PROBIOTICS:
HOW TO USE THEM
TO YOUR ADVANTAGE

PROBIOTICS:
HOW TO USE THEM TO YOUR ADVANTAGE

*Why You Probably Don't Have Enough Probiotics
And What You Can Do About It*

Jo A. Panyko, BS, MNT

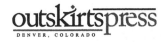

outskirtspress
DENVER, COLORADO

Disclaimer: The information contained in this book is educational in nature and is not intended as diagnosis, treatment, prescription or cure for any physical or mental disease, nor is it intended as a substitute for regular medical care. Consult with your doctor regarding any health or medical concerns you may have.

To Steve, the man of my life, for your never-ending love, support, humor and patience through all of our journeys together; and to Alison, Ellen and Alex, for being true blessings in my life.

Acknowledgments

Thank you to my husband and children for your unconditional love and unwavering support, and to my parents for introducing me to things I did not understand at the time.

Thank you to Shari Navarette, my lifelong friend, for your friendship and insightful editing suggestions.

Thank you to Alison Bailey for your talented editing suggestions.

Thank you to all of the researchers in the probiotics/microbiome realm for your meticulous work.

Finally, I am grateful to everyone who has touched my life and helped to make me the person I am.

Table of Contents

Introduction to the Concept of Probiotics

You are outnumbered. Resistance is futile. The microbes in and on your body outnumber your human cells, with some studies showing the ratio as being ten to one[1], depending on calculation methods. Additionally, microbial genes vastly outnumber human genes.

Seemingly unrelated health challenges such as weight gain, food poisoning, digestive and reflux issues, intestinal problems, vaginal issues, urinary problems, mental health and others have one thing in common: they all can be linked to these microbes.

Not all microbes are bad, however; there are beneficial microbes called *probiotics* which can actually help with health challenges!

This book focuses on:

- Why probiotics should fit into your life (including over 29 different benefits to you!)
- Why you probably do not have enough of them because of things you eat, take and do (things you do not even realize!)

- How you, the host, can strategically use your outnumbered status to your advantage, particularly in your gastrointestinal (GI) tract.

Although this book focuses primarily on the benefits of probiotics to your digestive tract, you will understand how probiotics may be beneficial for a wide range of conditions such as:

- Allergies
- Constipation, diarrhea, reflux (GERD), IBS (irritable bowel syndrome), IBD (irritable bowel disease) and pouchitis
- Reproductive challenges such as bacterial vaginosis, candidiasis and infertility
- High cholesterol and cardiovascular risks
- Urinary tract infections (UTI) and kidney disease
- Skin conditions such as eczema, acne and atopic dermatitis
- Mental health conditions such as anxiety and depression
- Arthritis and osteoporosis
- Pulmonary infections
- Obesity, diabetes and chronic fatigue syndrome
- Some cancers
- Improved athletic performance

The Quest for Answers

Learning about health has been and still is an exciting journey for me as an adult, but I did not think it was exciting when I was a child. My father did not allow junk food and sodas when I was growing up. For many years he had a massive garden and he and my mother jarred a lot of produce. We ate simple foods on a strict budget together as a family. I felt cheated compared to my friends who had access to junk food, and I loved going to their houses and having it. I had no idea what it was doing to my gastrointestinal tract, to my health and to me.

As a young adult, I developed numerous health problems and took multiple courses of antibiotics, mainly for sinus infections. When I became a mother, I wanted my children to be as healthy as possible and thus my quest for answers to questions about health began in earnest. Through my research, I gradually learned what nutrition meant and why my father was so adamant about it and about family dinners. I was able to solve the causes of my sinus infections, without antibiotics, and get autoimmunity under control.

Part of the solution to my health problems involved daily home-cooked family dinners and home-packed lunches in which I could control the ingredients. As a result, those were and are routine in our house. My kids have not-so-fond memories of being subjected to glop-like smoothies and various epic culinary failures. However, over time and with perseverance, I learned how to mesh flavor with nutrition and we began to enjoy tasty and nutritious, home-prepared food. Of course, an epic failure still occurs occasionally when I try new recipes!

My kids also remember me trying to sneak probiotic bead capsules into their yogurt or applesauce since they couldn't swallow them with water. Without understanding the intricacies of probiotics, I knew they had some kind of magical benefit. We have been using them in our family for over 20 years.

After years of employment as an engineer and then years of proper nutrition schooling, continuing education courses and my own zest for knowledge, I started my own business as a nutrition therapist with this keen interest in probiotics and anything having to do with digestive health. It is with this passion that I created the popular science-based, informational website, www.PowerOfProbiotics.com, and wrote this book, because I have learned how amazing and powerful probiotics truly are!

The concept of probiotics is simple, but the details are not. There is much misconception on blogs, websites and in the media about probiotics. I see it in my interactions with other healthcare professionals, with my nutrition clients, with people who contact me via my website, PowerOfProbiotics.com, and with the general population.

I have two goals in writing this book:

1. The first one is to dispel many of the misconceptions people have about probiotics. There is a lot of misinformation passed on by well-meaning folks!

2. The second one is to help you gain an understanding of probiotics so you can use them to your advantage to optimize your health. Probiotics offer many benefits to you which will become clearer as you read through the book. When you are faced with the incredible magnitude of information on probiotics on the internet and through news media, it is no wonder that you may feel overwhelmed and not know what to believe. It is not your fault!

While you may not be as enthusiastic about the details of probiotics as I am, I hope you will appreciate the essentiality of having them in your life.

Let's Begin with the Basics

Microbes are the microscopic bacteria, viruses, protists, archaea and fungi, such as yeasts, that inhabit you. Microbes make up your *microbiota*, your community of organisms. Sometimes the microbiota is called *flora*. This microbiota only comprises about 2-6 pounds of your body weight, yet is essential for your survival.[1]

The microbiota have more genes than you have human genes. Technically, the community of organisms is called the *microbiota* and the genes they contain are your *microbiome*, but sometimes the words are used in mainstream press synonymously. The actions of those genes affect your body locally and systemically (body-wide).

Scientists understand that human life is influenced for good and for bad by the human microbiome. Research on animals has shown that without beneficial microbes there cannot be long-term health[2]. That is why scientists involved in many projects around the world are actively searching for the beneficial microbes, the probiotics, which can improve human health. Since the outcomes of these projects will ultimately affect what is known about health, it is helpful to you to have an overview of what is happening with these various projects.

The Human Microbiome Project (HMP)[3] is one of several international efforts being undertaken to analyze the various microbe populations that live in and on our human bodies and to discover their potential roles in human health and disease. The first phase of this massive project investigated where different microbes live and hypothesized what functions they could potentially perform based on their genetic makeup.

The current phase of the HMP explores what functions these microbes *actually* perform under certain conditions and how those relate to health and disease. One major project focuses on microbes in the gut and the nose to determine how variations may trigger the development of diseases such as diabetes. Another major project examines how microbe populations interact with the body in inflammatory bowel diseases such as Crohn's and ulcerative colitis. A third project investigates the bacteria that live in the vagina and how they impact pregnancy and preterm birth.

Other projects are also underway. The American Gut Project[4] by the Human Food Project is currently surveying a diversity of subjects (all ages, both sexes, no exclusions). American Gut is an open-source, community-driven effort to characterize microbial diversity for US and international participants. American Gut takes a stool, saliva and/or skin sample which you provide, along with your answers to a detailed questionnaire and diet diary, to tell you what your most abundant microbes are and which ones you have more of compared to most people in the project. The detail is down to the genus level.

British Gut[5] is the same kind of project as the American one, but offers services intended for Europeans to save them costly international sample submission and shipment fees.

These international efforts are not a quick-turnaround projects since sequencing takes time and the labs are research labs, not commercial labs.

Additional international studies are in progress as well. The MyNewGut Project[6], which is funded by the EU and includes partners from 15 countries, is studying the influence of the gut microbiome on brain development and function and on diet-related diseases such as obesity, especially in childhood and adolescence. The Asian Microbiome Project[7] is comparing a diversity of subjects across 11 sites (all ages, both sexes, including a sub-focus on mothers and healthy children). An African Microbiome Project[7] has recently been proposed.

There are also privately-funded companies that will sequence your microbiota and I work with some of the laboratories that do.

These are exciting times in microbiome history!

Three common themes are emerging from these research projects:

1. The human gut microbiota and the microbial genome (microbiome) play diverse physiological roles that influence our health and wellbeing.

2. Particularly in the digestive tract, the less diverse the microbial community (and especially with harmful or opportunistic organisms dominating the flora), the less healthy the body can be.

3. Prevention of illness is easier than reaction to established illness.

Now that you know the very basics about probiotics and the fast pace of new research on them, it is time to find out how this book can help you.

The Advantage of Being Outnumbered – Finding a Strategy that Helps You Take Advantage of Probiotics

Here is what you will discover in this book about these three common themes and how you can use your outnumbered status from the human microbiome to your advantage. The information in this book is presented like a story, and each chapter builds on the information in the previous chapters. Although you might be tempted to skip to the later chapters, the beginning chapters will give you a solid foundation to better understand the later chapters.

Chapters 1, 2, and 3 and 4 explain what probiotics are, who benefits from them, how they are named, and where they live.

Chapter 5 summarizes how probiotics work.

Chapter 6 summarizes why you should take probiotics, how probiotics benefit your health and which microbes benefit some common digestive-system problems.

Chapter 7 explains why you probably don't have enough probiotics, including some critically important and surprising reasons.

Chapter 8 explains how to introduce probiotics into your daily life and what side effects may occur.

Chapter 9 outlines the major players in the probiotics world and their actions on the body.

Chapter 10 gives you resources on where to get probiotics and when to take them.

Chapter 11 details fourteen things to consider when buying probiotics products, including how to choose a probiotic supplement.

Chapter 12 provides summary recommendations and perspectives about probiotics.

Chapter 13 provides recipes and insights for you to begin enjoying fermented foods and drinks, probable sources of probiotics.

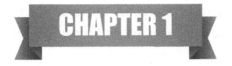

CHAPTER 1

What Are Probiotics?

Probiotic literally means "for life." Probiotics are officially defined by the Joint Food and Agriculture Organization (FAO) of the United Nations as, "**Live organisms that, when administered in adequate amounts, confer a health benefit on the host.**"[8] There are five categories of probiotics generally recognized in the industry:[9]

1. Probiotic supplements
2. Probiotic drugs
3. Probiotic foods
4. Direct-fed microbials for animal use
5. Designer, genetically-modified probiotics.

First, understand that the FAO definition was established to protect you when you are buying products with probiotics. Since this definition is important for you, the consumer, to understand, let's take a closer look at it.

"Live organisms…" Currently these organisms consist of certain bacteria and yeasts which, when in or on the body, perform certain functions or secrete specific chemicals. In order for them to perform those functions or secrete those chemicals, they have to be alive.

This **doesn't mean** that once the bacteria or yeasts are dead that they serve no beneficial purpose. Studies have shown that dead forms of some of those microbes CAN have positive effects on the body. In fact, even the culture in which the bacteria or yeasts were grown can have beneficial effects.[10]

However, when you the consumer are buying a product, you want the microbes to be alive so they can maximize the benefits they provide and possibly replicate and increase their numbers. More about this subject is provided in Chapter 11.

"…when administered in adequate amounts…" Some probiotics are required in numbers in the tens of billions in order to have a demonstrable effect on the human body. Others can be present in millions of microbes and have positive effects. Each type of microbe is different because each type of microbe acts differently. As a consumer, you want to make sure you are getting at least the minimum numbers of microbes that have been shown to produce positive effects for a given condition, and that's where a book like this one and a website like PowerOfProbiotics.com are helpful. Products advertising vague statements such as "contains probiotics" do not tell you if there are enough inside to make a difference for you.

"…confer a health benefit on the host": This is where the definition gets tricky. What exactly determines a health benefit has not been established for most probiotic products on the market and that is why most probiotic products cannot state specific health claims on their labels.

Probiotic products that have been approved for specific medical claims are classified as medical foods (in the US). The term medical food, as defined in section 5(b) of the Orphan Drug Act (21 U.S.C. 360ee (b) (3)) is "a food which is formulated to be consumed or administered enterally (*through the digestive tract*) under the supervision of a physician and which is intended for the specific dietary management of a disease or condition for which distinctive nutritional requirements, based on recognized scientific principles, are established by medical evaluation."[11] These medical foods are supposed to be used under a doctor's orders. In some cases, only the super-potent form is prescription-only (in the US). These probiotic drugs are by definition intended to treat, cure or prevent disease.

Most governmental regulatory agencies have not approved specific health claims for probiotic products and instead allow what are called *structure/function claims* such as "improves digestive and immune health". Similar claims are found on most other natural health products, too. These products are not proven to act like drugs and a result, cannot be labeled with specific disease health claims.

Health benefits of probiotics gleaned from scientific studies extend beyond the general structure/function claims in many instances and are discussed in Chapters 6 and 9. While these health benefits have not undergone regulatory approval, they nonetheless have been discovered and may be of use to you.

In addition to the official definition of probiotics from the FAO of the United Nations, ISAPP (International Scientific Association for Probiotics and Prebiotics), an international non-profit collaboration of scientists, recommends that fermented foods with undefined microbial content NOT be classified as probiotics unless they meet a specific criteria, such as the improvement of lactose digestion in lactose maldigesters. ISAPP also recommends that a probiotic have the strain designated for a specific health claim since many targeted actions are strain-specific.[12] Unfortunately, even those probiotics designated as medical foods may not disclose the strains.

What about colonization ability of these live organisms? Some manufacturers argue that probiotics must colonize the body and become part of the permanent flora in order to confer health benefits, but this is not true. While certain species of microbes do in fact colonize inside or on us, others have beneficial effects while passing through or by. These passers-by are known as *transient* microbes and they can positively (or negatively) affect our microbiome. Most of them lose their effectiveness if discontinued and are cleared by the body in about a week.

The summary of what does and doesn't qualify as a probiotic is this:

- Probiotics are alive.
- Probiotics are in adequate amounts.
- Probiotics should be defined at least at the genus and species levels for general claims and at the strain levels for specific health claims.
- Probiotics are safe for the generally healthy population.
- While not explicitly in the definition, many academic and industry scientists have stated that probiotics are not

supposed to have the capability to transfer or accept genes from other microbes. This protects people from taking microbes which may have the potential not only for antibiotic resistance, but also for toxin-production or virulence ability which can cause illness or even death.

- Probiotics may provide benefit to you.
- Probiotics may be part of your beneficial microbiota.

BUT not all beneficial microbes, even those in your flora or in products with "live, active cultures", are officially classified as probiotics.

Please note: Fecal enemas have shown great promise for *C. difficile* infections and IBD (irritable bowel disease) so far. While fecal enemas may contain probiotic species in them, at the current time those enemas are not specifically classified as probiotics.

Note that a new trend in probiotics is to include bacteriophages (phages), viruses that attack targeted *pathogenic* (disease-causing) bacteria, added to probiotic bacteria and/or yeasts. The rationale is that the probiotics and the phages can both exert positive influences to reduce pathogenic bacteria numbers. Phages are not officially considered to be probiotics, so in this book, only the actions of probiotic bacteria and yeasts are explored.

Another trend is to take specially-formulated prebiotic supplements either as stand-alone supplements or in combination with probiotics. Some information about this trend is provided in Chapter 11.

To learn how to use probiotics to your advantage, next you need to know who needs them.

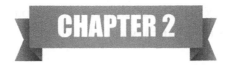

CHAPTER 2

Who Benefits from Probiotics?

Before you read about how probiotics are named, where they live, how they work, when to take them and how to choose them, you need the answer to an important question: Who benefits from probiotics?

The answer may surprise you: Every living creature needs beneficial microbes, although specific microbes vary among creatures. Yes, from the annoying mosquito to the laboratory mouse to livestock to your beloved pet to yourself, every living creature has some bacteria and other microbes in its gut and many of those are beneficial. As you learned previously, microbial cells and genes outnumber human cells and genes. However, microbes are small, only about one-twentieth to one-tenth the size of a human cell. Many of them can fit in a tiny space.

In the case of the mosquito, scientists found that bacteria in the mosquito's gastrointestinal (GI) tract offer health protection through different processes: stimulation of the mosquito immune response, competition for binding sites or nutrients and production of toxins.[13] These actions are similar to what occurs inside you as you will see in a later chapter. If gut bacteria can protect mosquitos, imagine what they can do for you!

In the case of livestock, probiotics are routinely used in animal feed to reduce infections and in some cases, accelerate weight gain. Poultry, swine, ruminants such as cattle, sheep and goats, and even farmed fish routinely are fed probiotics to maximize gut health and animal profitability while decreasing animal morbidity. Even the silage that many animals are fed is often treated with probiotics to minimize waste. The global probiotics animal feed market alone is projected to be worth 4.4 billion dollars by 2019![14]

In addition to probiotics in animal feed, liquid-encapsulated probiotics can be sprayed on baby chicks. When the chicks peck at and fluff their feathers, they ingest the probiotics and inoculate their guts with beneficial microbiota to help prevent dangerous *Salmonella* infections that can develop.

Pet food makers are also on the bandwagon to include probiotics in their products. Since upset stomach/vomiting and intestinal upset/diarrhea are among the top ten reasons why pets need veterinary attention[15], many of those episodes can potentially be avoided by keeping the pets' digestive tracts healthy with the help of probiotics. My dogs have been on probiotics for years and also get small amounts of fermented vegetables in their diet. While I cannot control what they eat or do every moment when they are in the backyard roaming free, I try to minimize any assaults on their health from what they ingest and therefore save money by avoiding vet visits.

As you can see, probiotics can benefit many different organisms, including you. Their widespread presence makes them a prime target for scientific research in genetic manipulation for treatment of disease. For example, scientists worked on a new way to attack the epidemic of malaria by genetically-altering the mosquito's gut bacteria. They discovered that the parasite that causes malaria is sensitive to proteins that one of the mosquito's gut bacteria has been engineered to produce.

Normally, this malaria parasite forms fertilized eggs with a thick-walled outer coating which can penetrate under the mosquito's gut lining. These eggs produce the long, worm-like organisms that swim into the mosquito's salivary glands and are deposited into the blood of whichever victim the mosquito bites. The proteins produced by the genetically-engineered bacteria are able to increase the resistance of the mosquito gut to penetration of these eggs and in some cases even kill them.[16]

Scientists are also looking at using genetically-modified bacteria in humans to diagnose, monitor and possibly even treat disease. Safety concerns regarding use of genetically-modified bacteria are valid concerns. The ethics and responsibility surrounding genetically-modified bacteria for use in living creatures is beyond the scope of this book, but I encourage you to learn about them and form your own opinion. Some information about herbicides used primarily on GMO (genetically-modified organism) plants is included in a later chapter.

Similar to many pharmaceutical studies, mice and rats are often used in probiotics studies. Although there is debate about the ethical use of animals in studies, there are several reasons why mice are the preferred subjects for many types of research. The most obvious are that mice have a small size, which makes them easy to handle, and short lifetimes, which makes it timely to see the effects.

Beyond the obvious, however, one of the reasons mice are used is that 99% of mouse genes have an equivalent in humans, and the mice can be genetically altered to have one particular gene substituted with the human equivalent. This makes it possible to study the effect of interventions on the "humanized" mouse. Not just any mice can be used in studies; there is a protocol for using specific mice or rats for specific studies so that data can be more standardized.[17]

Another lesser-known reason that mice are used in probiotics studies is that mice and humans share many of the same categories of intestinal bacteria.

Although specific microbes vary among creatures, the intestinal microbiota effects the health of each creature. So you see, humans are not alone in needing beneficial microbes in their gastrointestinal (GI) tracts! To decide which probiotic microbes you may want, you need to understand how microbes are named, and that is the topic of the next chapter.

CHAPTER 3

How to Understand What the Probiotic's Name Means

In biology, taxonomy is the science and practice of identifying, describing, naming and classifying organisms. Taxonomy is important because it shows the genetic lineage of organisms, which in turn shows which microbes are similar and which are not. Once you understand the lineage, you can understand at what level microbes are related and be able to ensure that you are getting the microbe you want.

The taxonomy of probiotics and other microbes can be compared to categories of recreational activity; this comparison is provided in Table 1. Following the table rows below, from top to bottom, using the probiotic *Lactobacillus acidophilus* DDS-1 as an example:

- Recreation is comparable to kingdom with the probiotic example of Eubacteria.

- The type of recreation (sports, reading, etc.) is comparable to phylum with the probiotic example of Firmicutes.

- For sports, the type of sport is comparable to class with the probiotic example of Bacilli, and so on, as shown below.

Note that the plural of phylum is phyla and the plural of genus is genera.

Table 1

Recreational Categories	Microbe Taxonomy	Probiotic Taxonomy
1. Recreation	1. Kingdom	1. Eubacteria (bacteria)
2. Sports, Reading, Gardening, Crafts	2. Phylum (Phyla)	2. Firmicutes
3. Type of sport: football, tennis, etc.	3. Class	3. Bacilli
4. Division conference	4. Order	4. Lactobacilliales
5. School	5. Family	5. Lactobacillaceae
6. Team	6. Genus (Genera)	6. *Lactobacillus*
7. Position	7. Species	7. *acidophilus*
8. Player	8. Strain	8. DDS-1

The major difference between the recreational categories and microbe/probiotic taxonomy examples are that all levels in the microbe and probiotic taxonomy columns (kingdom through strains) are genetically related. Just as any biological children you may have are related to you and you are related to your parents who are then related to their parents, and so on, taxonomy of microbes is like a family tree. So in this example, DDS-1 is the name of a strain of *Lactobacillus acidophilus* which is in the Lactobacillaceae family, the Lactobacilliales order, the Bacilli class, and the Firmicutes phylum in the Eubacteria kingdom.

The Firmicutes phylum is one of the three most common in the Westernized gut and is usually found in the highest proportion at approximately 60%. Bacteroidetes and Actinobacteria are the other two phyla comprising approximately 10% each.[18]

Probiotic microbes are named first by their genus (italicized), then by their species (italicized), and sometimes then by their strain, like this example: *Lactobacillus acidophilus* strain X. You may encounter the abbreviated versions of these names, such as *Lactobacillus acidophilus* X or *L. acidophilus* X instead of the full *Lactobacillus acidophilus* strain X name.[19]

One thing to be aware of so that you're sure you are getting the microbe you want is that there can be more than one species that is abbreviated with the same first letter. For example, *"L."* can mean *Lactobacillus* or *Lactococcus* (or any other *"L"* genus name), *"B."* can be *Bifidobacterium* or *Bacillus* or *Bacteroides* (or any other *"B"* genus name) and "S" can mean *Saccharomyces* or *Streptococcus* (or any other *"S"* genus name).

The genus includes a number of core genes common to all species in that genus. Likewise, every strain in each of those species has the same core genes, too. The differences lie in the variable genes which change between every species and every strain.

It is those variable genes which cause significant differences between microbes. Therefore, the effectiveness of probiotics, in many cases, is both strain-specific and condition-specific, because of those variable genes. For example, you cannot expect every strain in the *Lactobacillus rhamnosus* species to act identically because the minor differences in their genes make them act differently.

When I first started this journey, many years ago in my quest to understand probiotics, I thought I could buy a high-powered microscope and differentiate between the various microbes. After all, the different bacteria and yeasts have different physical characteristics: some are round; some are oblong; many cluster in chains; some cluster in bunches; and so on. I didn't understand then that the difference of a few genes down to the strain level can make different microbes have different functions. Those genetic differences cannot be seen through a microscope.

Although you, the consumer, are concerned about what particular species/strains are most effective for you, the majority of probiotic research in diseases and health is only narrowed down to the phylum level, or, at most, the species level. Researchers are looking at the bigger picture of microbe interactions, not at YOUR particular microbiome interactions, and generally, the more specific the study is, the more expensive it is.

Research on particular strains usually results in a patented product due to the time and expense involved in doing the research. An example of this is *Lactobacillus rhamnosus* strain GG. If *Lactobacillus rhamnosus* GG is proven to benefit a given condition, another *Lactobacillus rhamnosus* strain, Strain F for example, cannot be implied to have the same effects as GG. Likewise, an undesignated strain labeled only as *Lactobacillus rhamnosus* cannot be construed to be the same as GG.

Now you have a better understanding of how probiotics are classified and named, as well as why variable genes are so important. Knowing where certain microbes typically live can help guide you in your buying decisions and that is the subject of the next chapter.

CHAPTER 4

Where Do Probiotics Live?

Microscopic organisms are found in and on our bodies in major mucosal surfaces and on our skin. Mucosal surfaces are slick and slippery due to the mucus on them and include nasal passages, trachea/lungs, eye membranes, oral cavities (mouth and esophagus), gastrointestinal (GI) tracts and urogenital tracts.

The microbial communities (recall *microbiota*) reside in many parts of your body, and their relative populations differ depending on their location. Your colon, for example, has an intestinal flora that differs from the community found in your nasal passages. And although there are similarities in the communities between people, each person has their own unique microbiota which can even vary over time!

Although the microscopic organisms make up approximately 1-3% of your body's mass, they play a truly vital role in health. Microbes also contribute more genes that are critical for your survival than you have yourself. Estimates are that you have 360 times MORE microbial genes than human ones in/on your body.[20]

Since most probiotics (but not all of them) are taken into your body through your mouth and are prevalent throughout your gastrointestinal tract, this book focuses only on these GI tract probiotics and the gut microbiome. In the gut, estimates are that microbial genes outnumber human genes by approximately 150 times, and that each individual harbors at least 160 different bacterial species with bacterial numbers outnumbering or being equal to human cell numbers.[21,22]

I like to compare probiotics and other GI tract microbes to human society. They are very similar to human society in five ways:

1. Contributions
2. Variety
3. Interactions
4. Clustering
5. Transience

Contributions: In any successful society, the contributions of those that benefit the society must outweigh the negative influences of others. Those contributions must also be diverse enough to meet the needs of the society. In human societies, some people make great contributions; some don't do any significant good or harm and live a peaceful, neutral existence; some normally are peaceful but can end up looting if the opportunity presents itself; and some people act incorrigibly and do more harm than good.

A similar situation exists in the digestive tract. Many microbes are beneficial to the human or animal host; some are neutral (commensal); some are beneficial or neutral but can cause opportunistic infections if not kept in their proper environment or in proper numbers (opportunists); and others do harm every chance they get (strictly pathogenic). If there is not diversity in the contributions of the gut microbes, and particularly if negative influences from harmful or opportunistic organisms dominate, then the body will be less healthy than it could otherwise be.

Variety: Microbes are also similar to a human society in that it takes many different kinds to maintain balance. Just as some people are doctors, some are lawyers, some are mechanics, some are cosmetologists and others fill a variety of jobs, the microbes in and on you have a variety of different abilities and functions and work together to maintain a healthy ecological balance. The human gut microbiota and the microbial genome (microbiome) certainly do play diverse physiological roles that influence our health and wellbeing.

Interactions: Another similarity of your microbiota to human society is that it takes interactions to make a society. Scientists have shown that microbes acknowledge each other and communicate based on a concept called *quorum sensing*. In quorum sensing, bacteria use chemical and electrical signaling molecules to communicate with our cells and with each other and to determine microbe population density.[23]

Quorum sensing enables bacteria to coordinate their behavior for survival. Survival involves adaptation to availability of nutrients, defense against other microbes which may compete for the same nutrients and the ability to avoid potentially toxic compounds. Communication between different species may even occur.

Quorum sensing is very important for pathogenic (harmful) bacteria during infection of a host such as a human, animal or plant.

This ability of pathogens allows them to coordinate their attack and defenses against the host's immune response so they not only survive, but also thrive and establish an infection. Pathogenic microbes such as Group A *Streptococcus* can actually detect when your body is under stress and increase their assault.[24]

Scientists are working on ways to interrupt this ability of bacteria to communicate as a means to manipulate drug-resistant bacteria. Quorum-sensing inhibition (QSI) strategies work by interrupting the signal production and/or signal detection of the targeted bacteria or by degrading or modifying the signal itself. However, bacteria differ in the ways they produce, detect and degrade or inactivate the signals, so QSI has to be specific to the targeted bacteria. QSI may be one way to combat antibiotic-resistant bacteria.[25] More about the subject of antibiotic resistance is discussed in Chapter 7.

Clustering: Another commonality between humans and microbes is clustering, in which organisms group together to live. Clustering provides protection, sharing of resources and companionship. When most people think about bacteria they think about individual bacterial cells that can be seen through a microscope. These individual cells are called *planktonic* bacteria, but they are not the way most bacteria are found in/on the body. Most microbes cluster together in pairs, chains, clusters and on surfaces in what are called *biofilms*.

Biofilms are essentially slimy masses of microbes attached to some sort of surface (like your intestines) with channels running through them. The channels allow the microbes on the inside of the biofilm to be protected yet still receive nutrients and have wastes removed. Microbes in the biofilms produce polysaccharides (long-chain carbohydrates), proteins and special molecules which form the matrix of the films. Biofilms make curing some infections particularly difficult because antibiotics target the individual cell, not the biofilm.

Examples of biofilms are dental plaque (which is why you have to brush your teeth to remove the plaque and not just rinse your mouth), middle ear infections, drain clog slime, slippery rock slime and shower scum. Estimates are that over 80% of microbial infections in the body are caused by bacteria growing as biofilms.[26]

According to a recent study[27], biofilms can be found on most colon polyps and cancers, especially those found on the right side of the colon. It is possible that by examining for the presence of biofilms via a noninvasive test, doctors may someday be able to predict which patients are most likely to develop colon cancer.

Biofilms containing probiotics like *Bifidobacterium* and *Lactobacillus* are mostly protective to us.

Transience: A final commonality that microbes share with human society is transience. Transient people pass from place to place, never establishing themselves in one location. When we go on vacations or holidays, we are just visiting the places we go and then we return home, so we are transient then. If we use our vacation time to do charitable work, then we are temporarily benefitting the societies we help. Some microbes are transient through our bodies and help us while they pass through, just like our charitable work, even if the microbes do not colonize us.

On the flip side, we can do harm when we travel through places by littering, defacing property, trampling on alpine growth and contaminating the water, among other things. Likewise, some microbes, such as those that cause food poisoning, can cause us harm when they pass through.

You can see that your microbes are very similar to human society in contributions, variety, interactions, clustering and transience. Just as the saying goes that it takes a village to raise emotionally healthy children, it takes a village of microbes to maintain a physically, mentally and emotionally healthy you!

Where Does This GI Village Exist and Who Is in It?

Many probiotic supplements are advertised for colon health, so it is logical to think that probiotics live in the colon. However, in your digestive system, probiotic microbes live in more places than your colon, such as in your mouth, esophagus, stomach, small intestine, and appendix. Each environment is suited for certain types of microbes, so each environment has unique types and numbers of microbes and these may vary depending of your age, stage of life (including pregnancy and lactation) and your diet.

To determine which microbes are present in the GI tract, *biopsy* (collection of a small tissue sample) and stool analysis are typically used. In the past, biopsy and stool samples were cultured to see what would grow and then the organisms were identified based on laboratory analysis. Some organisms grow well under these conditions, especially the *aerobic* (oxygen-dependent) microbes. Other microbes, such as many of the probiotic microbes, do not grow well in cultures because they are *anaerobic* (grow in the absence of oxygen). Even when culturing conditions were controlled for air content, culturing still favored some organisms over others. Modern identification techniques employ culture-independent techniques which help identify microorganism components but do not necessarily reflect the quantities of the microbes.

Culture-independent techniques such as fluorescence microscopy, bacterial microarrays, 16S rRNA/18S rRNA gene sequencing and metagenomics have significantly expanded scientific knowledge of the human microbiome. Nonetheless, realize that one method, be it culture-dependent or culture-independent, is not the be-all-end-all final word on what is really in our guts. The use of several methods in a study helps to more-specifically identify microbes, identify if they are capable of living and quantify them. Even with several diagnostic methods, microbes that do not fit in any predefined category are often encountered in gut sequencing and grouped into an unclassified category. This shows that there is much to learn about the gut microbiota!

In general, culture-independent techniques have shown that among healthy individuals there is:

- A high diversity of microbial types present in each individual
- Site-specific clustering of microbes with specific bacterial populations commonly found in specific areas
- Uniqueness per individual at the lower levels (species/ strains) of taxonomy.

The advanced culture-independent technologies are showing us that, in addition to the discovery of microbes that do not fit in any existing category, some microbes previously named by culturing methods have to be re-classified based on DNA/RNA. Such reclassification can make following the trail of research on a particular microbe challenging.

The numbers and types of microbial communities shift along the length of the digestive tract, which is typically about 16 feet long in the average adult, starting with high numbers in the mouth, decreasing through the stomach and beginning of the small intestine, and increasing through the end of the small intestine and colon.

The living space for these microbial communities also varies depending on the portion of the digestive tract. In the past, based on cadavers or on relaxed tissue during surgery, it was estimated that the area of the GI (gastrointestinal tract) tract was about the size of a tennis court (600-1,000 square feet), but a recent study puts the estimate at approximately 350 square feet.[26] Of course, the exact length and surface area of your GI tract may differ from other people.

Of that area, approximately 3% involves the mouth, esophagus and stomach and 6.5% involves the colon. The rest is accounted for by the small intestine (91.5%). This is an important finding because the small intestine has many folds and protrusions (called *villi*) that allow maximum surface area for maximum absorption of nutrients. Any decrease in that area due to celiac disease, Crohn's disease or other digestive disorders results in less efficient nutrient absorption.

Typical numbers of microbes (bacteria and others) in each section of the GI tract are:[28-32]

- <u>Mouth</u>: There are approximately 100 million microbes per gram. It contains the most diversity.
- <u>Stomach</u>: Yes, your stomach has bacteria in it despite the stomach acid! There are up to 1 thousand bacterial cells/ gram.

- <u>Small intestine</u>: There are approximately 10 thousand bacterial cells/gram in the beginning of the small intestine, increasing up to 10-100 million/gram near the end.

- <u>Colon</u>: There are approximately 10 billion to 1 trillion bacterial cells/gram

- <u>Stool</u>: Some estimates are up to 1 trillion microbes per gram.

As to who exists in the microbial communities along the GI tract, a recent order-level bacterial RNA study[33] from biopsies and stool samples of 4 healthy Canadian individuals (2 males and 2 females) showed that 5 orders dominated out of 49 orders identified. Some bacteria could not be classified. These 5 orders were Lactobacilliales, Fusobacteriales, Clostridiales, Bacteriodales and small percentages of Bifidobacteriales. From the mouth to the colon to stool samples, major residents were from helpful (with beneficial actions), neutral (commensal), opportunistic and pathogenic microbes in each section of the digestive tract.

One important takeaway from the Canadian study is that although some bacterial orders/genera/species are small percentages of the total bacterial count, their small percentages can have drastic effects of being very helpful or very harmful. Therefore, it is best to keep the pathogenic or potentially opportunistic microbes under control. Beneficial microbes such as probiotics keep the contributions, variety, interactions, clustering and transience of the microbes in the GI tract in favor of the "good guys" in order to maintain GI health.

The Canadian study mentioned above (and some other studies) showed that the ratios of the types of bacteria in colon biopsy samples differed somewhat from those in stool samples despite their similar microbial concentrations; however, still other studies have shown a pretty good correlation between stool and biopsy bacterial types.[34-38]

Differences may be due to the locations of the biopsies along the GI tract, how the biopsies were processed, the type of culture-independent method and the number of sample reads. Also, stool can be a cumulative collection of microbes all along the GI tract, not specifically at one segment.

If you've never collected a stool sample before, you need to realize that only a tiny amount of stool is actually sampled and that it is a snapshot in time. Human feces usually are made up of approximately 75% water and 25% solid matter. In the solid matter, about 30% to 50% is bacteria.[39] That tiny amount of stool sample may or may not be completely representative in absolute numbers or types of which exact microbes are throughout the GI tract or along the intestinal walls.

Likewise, biopsy samples are only small representations, too. **However, if stool analysis or biopsy shows that pathogenic microbe amounts are higher than they should be and probiotic species are lower than they should be, that means that a person most likely has *dysbiosis* (unbalanced microbiota) and an intervention with probiotics may be helpful.**

Now that you see where bacteria may live inside the gastrointestinal tract, how an intervention with probiotics may work to rebalance your microbiome is the subject of the next chapter.

CHAPTER 5

How Do Probiotics Work?

Now that you know what probiotics are, who benefits from them, how they are named and where they live, the next logical step in learning how to use them to your advantage is to understand an overview of how they work.

In short, probiotics work by significantly impacting your digestive, immune, nervous and endocrine systems and their functions, as well as other bodily functions, in beneficial ways, whereas not all species in your flora do. More about some of the dangers of harmful bacteria and how probiotics can mitigate them are in the next chapter. As you will see in the next chapter, probiotics can also affect every system in the body. Most of those effects probably have their origins in either the digestive, immune, nervous or endocrine systems.

The Probiotics to Digestive and Immune Systems Connection

First, let's look at your digestive and immune systems. Your digestive system takes the food and drinks you consume, breaks them down into useable components and absorbs them into your body for nourishment while subsequently eliminating wastes. Since probiotics reside in or pass through your digestive system, it makes sense that they could impact your GI tract. More information about how they do that is provided in the next chapter.

In your digestive tract, there is a sheet of epithelial (tissue) cells that line the tract and act as a barrier so that only desired substances are supposed to pass through to your bloodstream. These cells are meant to stay close together. On top of the epithelial cells in the digestive tract are mucus and microbes. The mucus is supposed to be thick and continuous in order to separate the epithelial cells from microbes and gut contents. In many GI conditions, the mucus is disrupted. Probiotics can affect mucus in positive ways as Chapter 6 shows.

Your immune system protects you from external invaders and internal abnormal cells. Underneath the epithelial cells in the digestive tract are immune cells generally referred to as *GALT*, or gut-associated lymphoid tissue. GALT is the largest lymphoid tissue of the body's immune system. Approximately 70-80% of your immune system is actually in your intestines! GALT is found in the intestines in organized patches and nodes as well as in scattered immune cells[40-42] and is very active in protecting your body.

As you might imagine, the epithelial cells lining your gastrointestinal tract (GI) tract can interact with and influence the GALT cells underlying them, forming an intricate relationship. Since the majority of your immune system is in your digestive tract, having an intact digestive system with those epithelial cells close together is very important to keep your immune system and your entire body healthy. An intact digestive tract also helps to prevent your body from mistaking your own tissue as being a foreign invader and mounting an autoimmune attack.

You may have heard of the term *leaky gut* which describes the presence of gaps in the junctions between the epithelial cells. With a leaky gut, your digestive system is compromised and it sets the stage for your immune system to react.

Fortunately, probiotics can help prevent leaky gut.

In their communication with the cells of your digestive and immune systems, probiotics influence, through chemical messengers, which genes are turned on or turned off. In turn, those cells communicate back. Thus, probiotics can affect how your genes and your *genome* (all the genetic material of an organism) work. This effect on genes can also determine how your immune system develops.[43]

You see, the genes you inherited do not necessarily determine your fate. If and how those genes are turned on or off is what matters. For example, there are many genes affecting Crohn's disease risk, and Crohn's disease is believed to be caused by an inappropriate response of the immune system. Even if you are genetically susceptible to Crohn's disease, estimates are that your risk of developing Crohn's based solely on having the genes is less than 30%. Estimates for ulcerative colitis and celiac disease are even lower.[44-48] Probiotics play a role in appropriate gene and immune responses.

Since my genes, my lifestyle factors and my environment are different from yours, it cannot be assumed that what affects my microbiome in one way will affect your microbiome in the same way. Even if we have common genes between us, the activation or deactivation of those genes can be dependent on our lifestyles and environments. By influencing our body environments, probiotics influence our genes and can serve as preventive measures for disease.[49]

That explains why data from the Human Microbiome Project shows that there isn't one specific type of gut microbiome associated with health; gut flora and genetics differ from person to person. Species that may predominate in one individual may be found in very low numbers or be completely absent in another. What seems to define health is that the actions of the beneficial microbes, including probiotics, overpower and either control, or completely eliminate, the pathogenic microbes.

The environment around your gut microbiome depends on diet and lifestyle. Although studies show your microbiome is relatively stable, changes from a different diet can start to be seen in the gastrointestinal tract in as little as 24 hours, even before the remains of the food has left the body.[50] These changes stop once the food is stopped. So by simply changing your diet, you can begin to change the relative makeup of your microbiota and the way those microbiota interact with you.

The Probiotics to Nervous System Connection

It is easy to see how probiotics can affect your immune system through your digestive system. But what is the probiotics to nervous system connection? Your nervous system consists of your brain and all of the nerves in your body. Your first brain is part of your central nervous system. However, it is less commonly known that your gut acts as a "second brain", functioning as your *enteric nervous system*. Both brains originate from the same fetal tissue and each communicates with the other via nerves and neurotransmitters or their precursors. The functions of both brains can be affected by probiotics.

Your digestive system and your brain are directly connected predominantly by a major nerve, the vagus nerve, which runs between the two. Communication through this nerve is two-way, from the brain to the gut and from the gut to the brain. Estimates are that about 90 percent of the fibers in the vagus nerve carry information from the gut to the brain and not the other way around![51,52] The microbes in your gut communicate with your "second brain" which then communicates with your brain-brain via the vagus nerve. The brains can also communicate via chemical messengers in the bloodstream. Consequently, what happens in the gut doesn't necessarily stay in the gut and can affect many aspects of brain functioning including emotions and clear thinking.

The gut microbes also communicate with your endocrine system.

The Probiotics to Endocrine System Connection

Your endocrine system is the system in your body responsible for controlling bodily functions through the release of hormones and hormone-like chemicals. *Hormones* are substances which are released in one part of the body but usually affect other parts of the body by attaching to certain cellular receptors. Examples of endocrine organs and their commonly known hormones are:

- Pancreas and insulin
- Adrenals and cortisol
- Ovaries and estrogen and progesterone
- Testicles and testosterone
- Thyroid and thyroid hormones

What you may not realize, however, is that you have endocrine cells in your intestines, and the hormone-like substances produced by them can be influenced by probiotics. Also, many hormones are eliminated through the intestines after being processed through the liver and their fate can be influenced by probiotics. Additionally, through methods still being investigated, probiotics have the capability of affecting your body-wide hormones.[53] The probiotics to endocrine system connection is an exciting new area of exploration!

Now you see how probiotics work by significantly impacting your digestive, immune, nervous and endocrine systems. Then, primarily from these four systems, probiotics can influence all other systems in the body. Such an influence is beneficial in many ways, as the next chapter explains.

CHAPTER 6

What Are the Benefits of Probiotics and Which Conditions Can Be Helped by Them?

From the overview in Chapter 5 of how probiotics work to influence bodily systems, we are now going to explore some of the specific benefits probiotics provide to your body. There are at least 29 ways in which probiotics help you! If you understand the benefits generally, then you can appreciate how advantageous it is maintain substantial quantities and varieties in you.

As I mentioned in a previous chapter, the numbers and types of microbes vary along the gastrointestinal tract (GI) tract and from person to person. Some of those microbes are known as Gram-negative bacteria, some are Gram-positive bacteria, some are Gram-neutral bacteria, some are fungi/yeasts, many are archaea, a percentage are viruses and protists and all are part of a normal flora.

Official probiotics, which are mostly Gram-positive bacteria except for the Gram-negative *E. coli Nissle* and certain yeasts (and potentially *F. prausnitzii* in the future), impact your digestive, immune, nervous and endocrine systems and their functions in beneficial ways as explained in the last chapter, whereas not all species in your flora do.

What does this *Gram* designation mean? Hans Christian Gram was a scientist who developed a method of staining bacteria to make them visible in tissue samples. Over time, it became a way to identify the general type of bacteria quickly based on how the cell walls colored, as Gram-positive bacteria stain differently than Gram-negative ones.

Scientists estimate that bacteria evolved into Gram-negative and Gram-positive groups about one billion years ago.[54] However, not all bacteria stain either positive or negative consistently, and some don't stain at all, so that is where culture-free (fluorescence microscopy, bacterial microarrays, 16S rRNA/18S rRNA gene sequencing and metagenomics) analysis is particularly useful in identification of microbes.

What's the big deal with these Gram designations? The big deal is that Gram-negative bacteria have what is called *LPS* (lipopolysaccharides) in their cell walls which can cause major problems for us. The LPS of some bacterial species acts like a toxin in our bodies causing an immune response and even septic shock, a severe infection which can cause multiple organ failure and possible death.

LPS is often associated with different kinds of infections depending on the bacteria involved and is particularly hazardous if it enters the bloodstream via a leaky gut or via overwhelmed, normal body absorption processes. A leaky gut is one scenario in which the normal protective barrier (the intestinal wall) in the body is broken. This broken barrier allows particles, such as food molecules, LPS and bacteria, which would normally be prevented from entering the body tissues and bloodstream, to enter and cause problems. Since LPS from the Gram-negative bacteria causes an immune response, it leads to acute or chronic inflammation, even if it doesn't cause a significant, specific infection. Prevention of illness by keeping the gut lining intact is easier to manage than reaction to an established illness caused by a leaky gut.

Examples of pathogenic Gram-negative bacteria and the infections they cause are:

- *E. coli* (such as *E. coli* O157:H7, an enterohemorrhagic food-borne infectious strain which causes diarrhea, hemorrhagic colitis and hemolytic uremic syndrome)

- *Klebsiella* (such as *Klebsiella pneumonia* which can cause destructive changes to the lungs)

- *Salmonella* (such as *Salmonella enterica* which can cause food poisoning with symptoms of diarrhea, fever, abdominal cramps and occasionally cause localized infection or an infection in the blood)

- *Pseudomonas* (such as *Pseudomonas aeruginosa* which is an opportunistic bacterium that can cause infections of the blood, pneumonia and post-surgical infections, especially in people with weakened immune systems)

- *Legionella* (such as *Legionella pneumophila* which causes Legionnaire's disease)

- *Shigella* (such as *Shigella dysenteriae* which causes severe gastrointestinal distress)

- *Vibrio* (such as *Vibrio cholera*, a cause of cholera)

- *Neisseria* (such as *Neisseria gonorrhoeae* which is responsible for the sexually-transmitted disease (STD) gonorrhea)

- *Prevotella* (such as *Prevotella dentalis*, a common cause of dental infections)

- *Fusobacterium* (such as *Fusobacterium nucleatum* which is a very potent bacterium responsible for infections ranging from periodontal disease to invasive infections of the head, neck, chest, lung, liver and abdomen)

- *Bacteroides* (such as *Bacteroides fragilis*, one of the highly opportunistic members of the *Bacteroides* genus which is found with a high frequency in clinical infections and resistance to antimicrobial agents)

Many of these infectious Gram-negative bacteria are resistant to antibiotics so treatment can be difficult, especially if they are in biofilms.[55]

Note that not all Gram-negative bacteria cause infections, and likewise not all infections are caused by Gram-negative bacteria. Some species of Gram-positive bacteria such as *Streptococcus, Staphylococcus, Listeria, Bacillus* and *Clostridium* have strains which can also cause disease. Bacteria without cell walls, such as *Mycoplasma*, can also cause infections. However, LPS from Gram-negative bacteria is a known health hazard.

Many Gram-negative bacteria also have the capability of sharing their antibiotic-resistant genes with other bacteria via gene transfer, which you will remember from Chapter 1 is one trait that probiotics should NOT have. Additionally, several Gram-negative bacteria produce very toxic compounds with high biologic activity as well as enzymes which break down human tissue and immune-system molecules, thereby allowing their infections to spread more easily.[56]

Although Gram-negative, Gram-positive, Gram-neutral and cell wall-deficient bacteria can cause infections and be resistant to antibiotics, Gram-negative bacteria are significantly harder to kill due to the outer membrane of the cell wall. This outer membrane contains the LPS and is particularly adept at preventing certain drugs and antibiotics from entering the cell and killing it. To add to the pathogenic potential of harmful Gram-negative bacteria, it is now known that LPS from Gram-negative bacteria can coat viruses and protect them from your immune system,[57] which makes it harder for your immune system to detect, confront and eliminate viruses.

As you can imagine, LPS toxin in the bloodstream has the potential to affect every part of the body and cause inflammation. One huge benefit of probiotics, in general, is their ability to reduce or eliminate the bacteria that produce the LPS toxin. This one benefit alone can be very significant in health! Probiotics reduce the LPS-producing bacteria and protect against pathogenic (disease-causing) microbes, viruses and parasites inside you such as the food poisoning *E. coli* H0157:H7, *Candida* yeast overgrowth, and the other harmful microbes mentioned above. This occurs by several beneficial mechanisms, including the following:[58-66]

1. Crowding out the pathogens so there is no space for them to attach to tissues

2. Making it hard for pathogens to attach to your tissues

3. Displacing the pathogens from their attachment to your tissues

4. Making the environment too acidic for pathogens to survive by producing acids such as lactic acid or acetic acid, for example

5. Producing antibacterial/antifungal substances that kill pathogens. (Some of these probiotic antibacterial substances are even used in the food industry as preservatives!)

6. Stimulating your body to produce more protective mucus, more antibodies in that mucus, more white blood cells and more antibacterial substances to limit an infection

7. Helping your body decide if something is a friend or a foe

8. Affecting your bile acids so they are more toxic to pathogens

In addition to these 8 important benefits to you in reducing pathogenic microbes, and the very significant benefit of LPS reduction, probiotics have many other benefits. Some of these are listed below.

21 Other Benefits of Probiotics

Here are some other benefits of probiotics:[66-80]

1. Aid in digestion and nutrient absorption of humanly-digestible foods. Probiotics can digest sugars and other carbohydrates, which can help with problems such as lactose intolerance. Others degrade proteins in the colon so that the proteins do not putrefy there. Some can break down anti-nutrients, like phytates, in foods to make minerals more available to us.

2. Convert some plant compounds into active, beneficial forms that our bodies can use.

3. Provide energy for you from foodstuff you otherwise could not digest: Many complex sugars and fibers would pass through us and be useless to us without our microbes.

4. Play a role in the proper development and functioning of the intestines: Studies show that without proper flora the intestines do not develop properly.

5. Communicate with your body for proper development of your immune system: Studies also show that without proper flora the immune system is not primed properly and has dysfunctions.

6. Create a lasting benefit in several aspects of natural (innate) immunity and acquired (antibody) immunity: Our microbes can help prevent an over-exaggerated immune response to harmless substances and provide a competent response to harmful assaults from bacteria, yeasts, molds, viruses, and parasites.

7. Communicate with your genome: As I mentioned before, it is not only the genes you have that may determine your fate but how those genes respond to the environment around them. An intestinal environment full of pathogenic microbes will respond differently than it would if it were balanced with beneficial microbes.

8. Prevent leaky gut by helping your body's intestinal cells stay closer together: Tight junctions in the intestines are supposed to prevent rogue molecules from passing into the bloodstream. Probiotics affect those tight junctions in a positive way and thus can prevent immune responses and infections.

9. Communicate with your body's tissue cells to produce an

anti-inflammatory or pro-inflammatory response that can extend beyond the GI tract to other body tissues: Unlike Las Vegas, what happens in the gut does not necessarily stay in the gut. Both pro-inflammatory and anti-inflammatory molecules can leave the gut and influence tissues anywhere in the body.

10. Help to maintain the pro- to anti-inflammatory ratio of the immune system: Balance in the immune system is important to health. Different probiotics can affect the production of inflammatory and/or anti-inflammatory cytokines (chemical messengers).

11. Communicate with and/or influence other bacteria to perform functions they otherwise would not do.

12. Produce short-chain fatty acids (SCFA's) that nourish your colon cells and increase nutrient absorption.

13. Balance water and electrolyte absorption.

14. Balance your blood lipids.

15. Affect the metabolism of some drugs by enhancing their bioavailability.

16. Produce B vitamins and vitamin K for you or influence other bacteria which do.

17. Help your bowel movements to be regular, especially in diarrhea, constipation, IBS and other digestive disorders.

18. Re-populate the digestive tract quickly when consumed after you take antibiotics so that the harmful microbes don't become the majority.

19. Influence your behavior and moods (via the brain-second brain connection), as shown in Chapter 5.

20. Reduce other intestinal-derived toxins besides LPS that

may be carried in circulation and distributed to distant sites in the body.

The Benefits Keep On Going

Due to the benefits which probiotics can provide, it is no surprise that they can be helpful for many conditions, both within and outside of the digestive tract. Some of the different body systems and the conditions investigated with probiotics are:

- Immune system (autoimmune connection, allergies, possible HIV transmission prevention)
- Digestive system (food poisoning, constipation, diarrhea, reflux [GERD], IBS, IBD)
- Reproductive system (bacterial vaginosis, candidiasis, infertility, herpes simplex 2 virus)
- Cardiovascular system (atherosclerosis)
- Excretory system (kidney disease, UTI)
- Integumentary system (eczema, acne, atopic dermatitis)
- Nervous system (anxiety, depression)
- Skeletomuscular system (arthritis, osteoporosis)
- Respiratory system (pulmonary infections, cystic fibrosis pulmonary deterioration, respiratory tract infections)
- Endocrine system (chronic fatigue syndrome, obesity, diabetes)
- Global disease states such as some cancers
- Improved athletic performance

Probiotics can influence many of these bodily systems and

conditions through the 29 benefits you discovered earlier in this chapter. However, recognize that many of the benefits, despite how significant they can be, are not commercializable in the US. Many of them contribute to improved overall health, unlike drugs, which target diseased body segments.

Unless a probiotic goes through the drug-approval process to benefit a specific disease, which requires large sums of money and time, a probiotic product can only state a structure/function claim as you saw in Chapter 1. Therefore, although any single benefit, such as #13 above (water/electrolyte balance), could improve your entire body, it has not been shown to treat or cure some disease or one that has been singled out as a marketable trait. As a result, you will not see research, beginning with in-house laboratory petri dishes, then to genome sequencing, and progressing to animal studies, then to human studies and finally to full-blown clinical trials, on a probiotic marketed to balance water and electrolyte absorption. That does not diminish the importance of what that probiotic can do for you, however.

Keeping that in mind, there are some probiotics that *have* been studied in the hopes of improving some particular medical condition. Some of them are classified as medical drugs, many are patented for their actions, but most of them still retain only the structure/function claims.

Some of the probiotics I have listed below are not even on the market yet with any structure/function claims. I have listed them only to show you that there is the potential for a particular microbe, or several microbes, to have effects on bodily functions significantly enough to possibly benefit you for certain conditions.

Let's look at a few gastrointestinal conditions you may be struggling with and see which specific types of microbes have been investigated at some level for helping those conditions. More information about each of the major probiotic genera and species is provided in Chapter 9. Information about other conditions is available on my website, www.powerofprobiotics.com.

Note that I am not diagnosing, prescribing, treating or curing any condition, be it mental or physical. If you suffer from any of these conditions, you can research many of the details further and discuss them with your preferred medical professional. Note also that some conditions present differently in children versus adults, so that what might help in one group may be ineffective in the other. Lastly, these short lists are not all-inclusive.

Constipation

To aid in constipation, probiotics can play a role in the proper development and functionality of the intestines, balance water and electrolyte absorption and help with regularity.

In general, probiotics work best as preventive agents, not as quick "cures". But many times probiotics can help with constipation once it is an established condition.

Some probiotics that have shown efficacy in helping constipation are:[81-83]

- *E. coli* Nissle 1917 (adults, 25 billion CFU/day)
- *Lactobacillus casei* Shirota (adults, 6.5 billion CFU/day)

- *Bifidobacterium lactis* DN-173010 (adults, 150 million to 1.5 billion CFU/day)

- *Lactobacillus rhamnosus* Lcr35 (children, 800 million CFU/day)

Diarrhea

In various cases of diarrhea, probiotics can contribute similar aid as they do for constipation. Probiotics also competitively exclude the pathogenic microbes causing the diarrhea by methods previously mentioned, preserve gut-barrier function and recruit immune–system involvement, among other functions.

Specifically, probiotics have been shown to:[84-87]

- Prevent antibiotic-associated diarrhea. Some examples are:
  * *Lactobacillus acidophilus* CL1285 and *Lactobacillus casei* LBC80R (adults, 50-100 billion CFU/day))
  * *Lactobacillus casei* DN-114-001, *Lactobacillus bulgaricus* and *Streptococcus thermophilus* (adults, 420 million CFU/day)
  * *Lactobacillus acidophilus* CL1285 and *Lactobacillus casei* (adults, 50 billion CFU/day)
  * *Saccharomyces boulardii* (Adults, 30 billion CFU/day)
- Help in treatment and prevention of rotavirus diarrhea in children. Some examples are:
  * *Saccharomyces boulardii* (80 billion CFU/day)
  * *Lactobacillus acidophilus*, *Lactobacillus rhamnosus*, *Bifidobacterium longum* and *Saccharomyces*

boulardii (250 million CFU/day)

 * *Lactobacillus rhamnosus* GG (1-100 billion CFU/day)

- Help in treatment of relapsing *Clostridium difficile* diarrhea. A few examples in animals are:

 * *Lactobacillus rhamnosus* GG

 * *Saccharomyces boulardii*

 * *Bacillus coagulans* GBI-30, 6086

- Help prevent acute diarrhea and traveler's diarrhea.

 * Many probiotics can help with this since most of these infections are caused by a disturbance in gut flora

Reflux (GERD)

Balancing the gut flora and encouraging proper functioning of the digestive tract are where probiotics excel, so it shouldn't be a surprise that probiotics may help GERD. Probiotics work on the root cause of some forms of GERD, not just the symptoms.

Treating the symptoms of a condition like GERD are what many medications do. For example, the goal of conventional anti-acid medications is to reduce stomach acidity. That can provide relief for the discomfort of excess stomach acid for the short-term and can be extremely beneficial for GERD that erodes the esophagus. Reducing the pH in the stomach may, however, hinder proper digestion and set the stage for dysbiosis (unbalanced flora) in the gastrointestinal (GI) tract with resulting conditions such as *SIBO* (small intestine bacterial overgrowth).

Some probiotics that have been specifically studied for GERD relief are:[88,89]

- *Lactobacillus reuteri* DSM 17938 (regurgitation in infants)
- *Bifidobacterium infantis* 35624 (adult pilot study)
- *Lactobacillus rhamnosus* GG (adult pilot study)

IBS-D (diarrhea-predominant irritable bowel syndrome), IBD-UC (irritable bowel disease, ulcerative colitis) Remission and Pouchitis Remission[90-92]

- The honor of benefitting all three of these conditions goes to the multi-species, medical grade probiotic supplement, VSL#3. A review of the product is on my website. Since it is a medical food, it can advertise its use for specific medical conditions.

- *E. coli* Nissle 1917 was efficacious in IBS in adults (2.5-25 billion CFU/day)

- *Bifidobacterium infantis* 35624 was helpful in IBS in women (100 million CFU/day)

- *Bacillus coagulans* GBI-30, 6086 preliminary data showed it was helpful for IBS.

Some Insights about the Benefits of Probiotics

One thing that's important to notice about the GI conditions above is that there wasn't just one particular probiotic species that was able to provide relief for one of them or all of them. There were many. This illustrates the concept that it takes a village of microbes to be healthy, and that what works for one person may not work for another because we are all unique individuals.

Another thing to note is that most of the time, improvement is not overnight. Although changes in microbiota can begin to occur fairly quickly (within 24 hours), it takes time to turn an unhealthy intestinal environment into a healthy one.

Additionally, keep in mind when reading articles about studies on microbes is that *in vitro* (in the laboratory petri dish) tests are useful to gain knowledge of strains and the probiotic effect and possible benefits, but the use of probiotics in human trials may give the best clue as to their usefulness in a given health condition.

Also, remember that each probiotic strain has its own specific properties, so any health benefits attributed to one particular strain cannot be assumed to be attributed to other strains, even strains in the same species.

Since probiotics and beneficial bacteria and yeasts are so important, why is that you probably do not have enough? The answer to that question is explored in the next chapter.

CHAPTER 7

Why Don't You Have Enough Probiotics and Beneficial Microbes?

You now know what probiotics are, who benefits from them, how they are named, where they live, how they work and the numerous benefits they can provide. You also know that probiotics are critical for health, yet why don't you have enough? There are many reasons for insufficient levels of probiotics and beneficial microbes in your GI tract and some of them include:

- Modern day diets
- Sugars
- Artificial sweeteners
- Diabetes and sugar dysregulation
- Prescription and over-the-counter medication use

- Glyphosate, the active ingredient in herbicides such as RoundUp
- Disconnect of modern medicine to the concept of a whole body
- Lack of adequate sleep
- Stress

Understanding these reasons will help you determine positive changes you can make to support the numbers and types of beneficial flora in your body.

Note that this list is not meant to be fully comprehensive, but instead is meant to get you thinking about the effects on your microbiota of things you put in or do to your body. A good rule of thumb when considering things you put in or on your body is this: if something is not naturally found in nature in a particular form, then maybe it should not be in or on you.

Let's take a look at each of these reasons in more detail.

Modern-Day Diets

Food fermentation is a method of food preservation. Bacteria and yeasts transform sugars and starches in food into acids (such as lactic acid), gases or alcohol which then act to kill harmful microbes and preserve the food. As they preserve the food, the beneficial microbes increase in numbers as the pathogenic ones decrease. Many of the bacteria which ferment food are known to be probiotics. More information about fermented foods and drinks is provided in Chapters 10 and 13.

In the history of the human race, people hunted and gathered their food and ate what was in season for their particular part of the world. Together with drying and salting, food fermentation is one of the oldest methods of food preservation. It has been confirmed that over 9,000 years ago people drank fermented drinks.[93]

In human history, food and drink fermentation was a household- or village-level practice to preserve food, give food more flavor and reduce food toxicity. Many indigenous peoples around the globe, especially in East Asia and Africa, still consume fermented foodstuffs. In some cases such as mahewu, a fermented maize meal in South Africa, these fermented foods are staples in the diets of those people.[94]

In today's modern society, with the emphasis on industrial-scale food production and fast food, many of the old ways have been abandoned. Even in countries where fermented foodstuffs are still commonly prepared and still could serve as the basis of a healthy diet, the stigma that homemade fermented foods and drinks are only for the poor results in people abandoning them in order to purchase processed foods as soon as they can afford them.

Where did this stigma that homemade foods are only for the poor come from? Have advertisers' marketing distorted our perception of what is really valuable? More importantly, how do we dispel of that stigma? Homemade foods, including fermented foods, can be some of the most nutritious foods available made from simple ingredients that you can pronounce. These simple ingredients reset our taste buds to enjoy the subtle flavors the food offers in ways that experienced chefs know. When have you seen a world-renowned chef adding MSG, saccharin and other artificial sweeteners, artificial flavors and artificial colors to their dishes? You haven't, because real food doesn't need those things!

Modern people expect food to look appealing, taste sweet and/or fatty and/or salty and delicious and still expect to be able to go to a drive-through, pop food into a microwave oven or stop into a restaurant and have their food quickly available. Because of this, the modern-day diet is more heavily weighted towards questionable proteins and unhealthy fats and is scarce in fiber, vitamins, minerals, beneficial microbes and health-promoting plant compounds. We are fooled into thinking that because the quick "food" tastes good or satisfies our cravings (thanks to all the added chemicals manipulating our senses) that we are feeding ourselves. Instead, we are actually consuming things that take away from our bodies' stores of nutrients. Instead of nutrition, we consume only calories. There is a disconnect between "food" and nourishment.

Today's western societies focus on doing more in less time and for some aspects of life, that focus is appropriate. Modern appliances can certainly make our lives and food preparation easier. But to abandon the cultural ways of preparing and enjoying food together because we want to watch more television, go to more sports games or movies or go about our busy-ness is a mistake that is costing our society.

The Slow Food movement[95] that was started in Italy and is now an international movement is one effort to counter "the standardization of taste and culture" and preserve the "connections between plate, planet, people, politics and culture."

The Weston A. Price Foundation[96] is another effort at raising awareness about how our disconnect with the food we eat is affecting our health and the health of our planet. Part of their mission is "restoring nutrient-dense food to the human diet" and it emphasizes the importance of fermented vegetables, fruits, dairy, beverages and condiments in the diet.

Initiatives such as these are important, and if for nothing else than your personal well-being, I urge you to consider re-evaluating your diet and lifestyle and making nutritious food more of a priority in your life because modern processed food is void of the nutrients your body and your microbiota need in order to be healthy.

Modern food is typically very high in sugars, sodium, artificial flavors, artificial sweeteners, artificial colors, artificial preservatives, fake fats, stabilizers, emulsifiers and other ingredients which are, among other things, low in the nutrients (vitamins, minerals, essential fatty acids, phytochemicals) and fibers that feed the beneficial microbiota in your gut. Additionally, some of those very ingredients may be damaging to your beneficial gut microbes as you will see.

Sugars

Sugars can upset the ecological balance in your GI tract. Bacteria and yeasts of all types LOVE sugar as a food source. Since different microbes are able to reproduce at different rates, typically the microbes that should be absent or present in only small numbers (the harmful ones) reproduce faster than the beneficial microbes and take over when sugar is provided to them.

Sucrose, the regular sweetener simply called *sugar* that is obtained from sugar cane or sugar beets, is a 2-part sugar (a disaccharide) that is composed of the 2 one-sugar molecules (monosaccharides), glucose and fructose. Your body breaks down the sucrose into the monosaccharides.

Fructose, found predominantly in fruits and in small amounts in many vegetables (bound in the plant cells), is usually not a big problem until it is found in the form of free high-fructose corn syrup in processed foods and especially in soft drinks.

Combined, these 3 sugars (sucrose, glucose and fructose) are the simpler sugars which are used in most sweetened products and they are fuel for the growth of many microbes. Unfortunately, they fuel faster growth of undesirable bacteria and yeasts.

Salmonella, a bacterial species with many pathogens, thrives on glucose and doubles its numbers every 20 minutes or so under the right conditions. That is why infection symptoms can appear within 6-72 hours of infection. Also, *Salmonella* can make its own proteins to produce whip-like tails called *flagella* when it needs them. The flagella allow it to move to the nutrient-rich layers of the intestinal lining and continue growth and reproduction.[97,98]

In contrast, the doubling time of probiotic bacteria such as *Lactobacillus* or *Bifidobacterium* may be measured in HOURS or DAYS, not minutes, and many rely on you to consume the things to optimize their growth. Additionally, *Lactobacillus* and *Bifidobacterium* do not have flagella. So although probiotic microbes use glucose, too, they reproduce much more slowly, need more nutrients supplied from you than most pathogenic microbes do and are not able to propel themselves to the source of nutrients. Sugar intake puts the beneficial microbes at a disadvantage.[99,100]

Artificial Sweeteners

Okay, so you think you will do your microbiome a favor and skip the sugar and replace it with artificial sweeteners instead. Is that a good idea? From many health perspectives, including the risk of metabolic diseases and risk to the health of the beneficial microbes in your gut, that is not a good idea!

This book is focused on probiotics, so any information presented deals with effects of artificial sweeteners on the microbiota. However, I would be remiss if I did not mention that the general use of artificial sweeteners increases your risk for metabolic diseases such as obesity and diabetes.

The artificial sweeteners which have been studied for their effects on gut microbiota are:

- Saccharin (Sweet'N'Low)
- Aspartame (Nutrasweet, Equal)
- Sucralose (Splenda)

The results for all three show that they can modify bacterial communities in the GI tract, tipping the balance in favor of pathogenic microbes to the detriment of beneficial ones.[101-106]

What if you still want to use artificial sweeteners? Can taking probiotics be effective to prevent any bad effects on the gut microbiome from using them? That answer is not yet known. What is known is that the artificial sweeteners listed above increase your risk of a disrupted microbiota, among other conditions. Why would you still want to use them?

Diabetes and Sugar Dysregulation

Type 2 diabetes is a dysfunction in blood-sugar and insulin handling in the body causing abnormally high (and damaging) blood-sugar levels. Type 2 diabetes is primarily a result of poor diet and lifestyle. Type 1 diabetes is an autoimmune condition in which the person's immune cells attack and destroy the insulin-producing cells of the pancreas.

In the US alone, over 21 million children and adults, or over 9% of the population, has the diagnosis of diabetes. That is about 1 out of every 11 people and 90-95% of them have Type 2. Frighteningly, another 8 million-plus people have Type 2 diabetes and do not know it. That means that out of everyone with diabetes, almost one-third are undiagnosed and do not know it! Yet, on average, one American aged 20 and over is diagnosed with diabetes every 19 seconds. That equates to 4,660 people per day and 1.7 million per year.[107]

Even more frightening are the numbers of people who have pre-diabetes. Pre-diabetes means that blood-sugar levels are higher than normal, but not high enough to be officially diabetes. The CDC estimates the number of people with pre-diabetes to be more than 1 out of every 3 adults and 90% of them do not know they have it! For people who have pre-diabetes and do not lose weight and improve their diets and lifestyles, 15-30% will go on to develop full-blown diabetes. Pre-diabetes is a serious wake-up call to make immediate positive changes!

As you have seen from the information in this book so far, pathogenic microbes love sugars and they can easily use them to overpower beneficial microbes. And while the focus has been on sugars in the diet, which makes most people think only about the effects of the sugars in the digestive tract, those sugars in the digestive tract make their way into the bloodstream to cause high blood sugar levels there, too.

High blood sugar levels from any kind of blood-sugar dysregulation feed pathogenic microbes and encourage some harmful microbes, such as *Candida albicans*, to become invasive into our tissues. Invasive microbes are hard to displace.

So whether you have diabetes, pre-diabetes, or just sporadic high blood sugar levels from eating and drinking sugary and refined foods and drinks (candies, cookies, donuts, muffins, regular breads, boxed cereals, sweetened coffees, sodas, etc.), the net result to your microbiota is the same: You are favoring the pathogenic microbes and putting the beneficial ones at a disadvantage.

Prescription and Over-the-Counter Medication Use

Do you take medications? If so, you are certainly not alone. Nearly everyone in the Westernized world takes some kind of medication at some time. Statistics for over-the-counter medication use is not available, but in the US alone nearly 49% of people took at least one prescription drug during one month (2009-2012 statistics).[108]

During one month, nearly 22% of people took 3 or more prescription drugs and nearly 11% took 5 or more prescription drugs. Prescription drugs are big business and I don't need to tell you how expensive they can be. Over 260 billion dollars were spent in 2011 on those drugs in the US.

During doctor visits, over 75% of those visits to approximately 1500 physicians who answered a questionnaire in 2010 involved the prescribing of drug therapy. The most prescribed medications in those office visits were for pain, for high cholesterol and for antidepressants.

Besides contributing to many nutrient deficiencies, some prescription and over-the-counter (OTC) drugs have direct effects on gut microbes as you will see in the paragraphs below. These actions can be involved in the drug's side effects. Other drug actions have a more indirect, sneaky way of affecting your gut microbes in a bad way.

Interestingly, studies conducted back in the 1970's and to date showed that many medical drugs inhibit or kill human intestinal bacteria, including probiotic bacteria. Applying that knowledge, researchers are adding non-antibiotic medical drugs to antibiotic therapy to attempt to cure antibiotic-resistant bacterial infections.[109]

What is not being tested, however, presumably since there is no potential drug market involved, is what effect numerous drugs have on the probiotic bacteria within and on us.

In addition to blatant antibacterial activity, one of the sneaky ways that medications affect gut microbes is that many medications deplete nutrients. This makes it harder for the beneficial microbes, which need nutrients from us, to flourish. The classes and numbers of drugs that deplete nutrients is truly staggering.

For instance, birth control pills are known to deplete B vitamins, vitamin A, vitamin C, and many minerals.[98] Unfortunately, there are many microbes such as *Lactobacillus johnsonii* La-1 which rely on the host (that's you) or other microbes to provide it with nutrients for its basic needs, one of which is B vitamins. So birth control pills in essence rob you and your beneficial microbiota of nutrients for health.[110,111]

Additionally, while specific actions against the microbiota have not been investigated for most medications, **it is not hard to imagine that if the GI tract is affected by nausea, vomiting, constipation, diarrhea or general GI upset by any medication, whether over-the-counter or prescription, then there is the possibility that the microbiota is altered due to that effect.**

Let's take a look at four other popular types of medications which can adversely affect your microbiota: antibiotics, antidepressants, reflux drugs and NSAIDs.

Antibiotics

It is no secret that antibiotics kill life; that is their purpose. What is more of a secret is that probiotic bacteria take a serious death toll when antibiotics are used. Antibiotic-associated diarrhea (AAD) is one result.

Also, since antibiotics do not kill 100% of the bacteria, of the bacteria that remain, the harmful ones are able to quickly outnumber the beneficial ones, as was shown with the case of *Salmonella* in a previous chapter. **The result is a flora that may never fully recover to its previous health.**[112]

Some antibiotics are not marketed as antibiotics. For instance, an FDA-approved drug, Xifaxan (rifaximin), which was originally approved for treatment of travelers' diarrhea caused by *E. coli* and for adults with recurring brain/mood problems caused by an over-taxed liver, has recently been approved for treatment of IBS-D (irritable bowel syndrome, diarrhea-predominant). It is meant to improve abdominal pain and stool consistency, but people pre-scribed this drug for IBS-D may not really understand that it is an antibiotic. They do not know that it has broad-spectrum efficacy against anaerobic probiotic bacteria such as many lactobacilli.

They also may not understand that ironically, it can cause stress on the liver (which could be causing brain/mood distortions and other problems that it was initially prescribed to treat!)[113]

We may be unaware of how significantly we are exposed to anti-biotics, and how they negatively impact the beneficial microbes in our bodies. Some of these exposures are through:

- Antibiotic medicines we take for infections
- Antibiotics in drinking water from improperly disposed medications and from human wastes
- Antibiotics which are used extensively in convention-al *CAFO*'s (confined animal feeding operations) and which can be found in CAFO meat, fish, poultry and milk
- Antibiotics present in manure or waste water used on produce
- Antibiotics sprayed on certain fruit trees for pest control

Previous information in this book discussed antibiotic-resistant bacteria and the possibility of using QSI (quorum-sensing inter-ruption) to combat them. Antibiotic resistance is a real and seri-ous concern and occurs because some bacteria are able to adapt to threats on their existence. People die from infections because pathogenic bacteria develop resistance to even the most sophisticated antibiotics. Government agencies finally are realizing that measures to limit the use of antimicrobial drugs that are medically important for humans should be instituted, although some countries have been more proactive than others. Sadly, the US is not the leader in this effort.[114]

Note that although some probiotic bacteria naturally have resistance (intrinsic resistance) to one to three antibiotics, such as vancomycin, this resistance usually is part of their cell-wall composition. As such, the resistance is not genetically-transferable to other bacteria. Also, probiotic bacteria are usually susceptible to the most widely used antibiotics.

Research on antibiotic-resistance in different strains in different probiotic species is continuing and may show which ones are most susceptible to dangerous genetic exchanges. Probiotics that are comprehensively researched and genetically-sequenced should not have the capability to transfer mobile genetic elements containing antibiotic-resistant genes to other bacteria. Antibiotic resistance in sequenced probiotics should therefore be of a concern only when rare infections involving them are encountered.

What is the bottom line for consumers? Only use antibiotics when they truly are medically necessary, and never for a virus like a cold. Always take the full course of your antibiotics and never flush unused medications down the drain or in the toilet. Re-populate your GI tract with probiotics, potentially waiting 3 hours after taking each dose of antibiotic, if not contraindicated by your physician. Also, use your purchasing power to buy only those livestock, fish and poultry products, as well as produce, which do not employ antibiotics.

Antibiotic resistance can also be caused by herbicides such as glyphosate in RoundUp, as you will see.

Antidepressants

A recent study conducted by University of Michigan researchers has shown that people with major depression have a much greater risk of contracting a bacterial *C. difficile* infection than those without depression. *C. difficile* (*Clostridium difficile*) can cause life-threatening GI infections that are hard to cure. Taking either antidepressant, Remeron (mirtazapine) or Prozac (fluoxetine), DOUBLES the risk of a *C. difficile* infection, and taking both mirtazapine and trazodone (Desyrel) together increased the risk of a *C. difficile* infection by almost 6 times.[115]

Tests *in vitro* (in a laboratory dish) showed that the SSRI's (selective serotonin reuptake inhibitors) sertraline (Zoloft, Lustral), fluoxetine (Prozac, Sarafem) and paroxetine (Pexeva, Paxil) have significant antimicrobial activity, mainly against Gram-positive bacteria (which many probiotics are) yet are inactive against most of the Gram-negative bacteria (many of which are pathogenic as you saw in a previous chapter).[116]

Whether or not these results directly reflect what happens in the gut is unknown. However, a common side effect of SSRI's is gastrointestinal upset experienced as a wide range of symptoms from dry mouth to diarrhea. Such upset can be due to the effect of the serotonin receptors in the gut as well as the possible detrimental influence on the beneficial microbiota.

Antidepressants in water are another concern. Tiny concentrations of the antidepressant fluoxetine (Prozac) found in the Great Lakes of the US were found to kill off microbial populations of *E. coli* and *Enterococcus* bacteria in the water.[117] These species of bacteria contribute to the microbial society in your GI tract in ways discussed in Chapter 4. While they can cause infections when not kept under control (they are opportunistic), they usually live inside us and either benefit us or do not cause harm (commensal). The question remains to be answered about how those concentrations of fluoxetine in water affect beneficial bacteria within/on us and in the ecosystem. Medications of any sort should never be flushed down the toilet.

Reflux (GERD) drugs

The goal of reflux drugs is to reduce the acidity of the stomach, which normally can range from 1-3 and be buffered to 4 or so when filled with food. Normally stomach acid protects against pathogenic bacteria because although they have various sneaky ways of adjusting to hostile conditions, many cannot survive low pH.[118] Reflux drugs eliminate this protective mechanism, allowing pathogens to pass through the stomach into the rest of the digestive tract where they can exert their harmful functions.

Probiotic lactic-acid producing bacteria, however, are generally able to survive in low pH. Stomach acid, therefore, is designed to allow helpful bacteria through, yet kill pathogenic ones.

Consider this if you are regularly taking some kind of acid blocker or neutralizer: laboratory animals are often given acid-blocking medications prior to the administration of pathogenic microbes so that the pathogens can become established in the GI tracts of the animals and the effects from the pathogens can be seen.

NSAIDS

It is a well-established fact that *NSAIDs* (non-steroidal anti-in-flammatory drugs) can damage the upper GI tract, the small intestine and the colon in many ways causing increased mucosal permeability, inflammation, erosions, ulceration, and even other more serious clinical outcomes such as anemia, and overall bleeding, perforation, obstruction, diverticulitis and deaths.[119]

NSAIDs are responsible for a marked reduction of lactobacilli. Other research has implicated NSAIDs in promoting the progression of bacterial infections by reducing the body's immunologic response to those infections. Recent research suggests that Gram-negative bacteria appear to be particularly important in the initiation and progression of NSAID enteropathy (disease of the intestines), possibly through release of LPS toxin.[120-122] As you saw in the last chapter, probiotics can reduce the microbes which produce LPS toxin.

Treatment with probiotics has shown promising positive effects against NSAID enteropathy in animal models with the beneficial effects believed to be due to colonization by the bacteria. There have also been human studies demonstrating preventive effects of probiotics against NSAID-induced small intestinal injury. Perhaps future research will shed more light on the exact mechanisms involved.

Glyphosate, the Active Ingredient in Herbicides Such as RoundUp

Glyphosate is the active ingredient in the herbicide, RoundUp. The chemical Roundup combines glyphosate with surfactants and other ingredients that make it easier for the glyphosate to get into cells. Glyphosate-resistant genetic material is used in GMO crops such as Roundup Ready corn, cottonseed, canola, soy, sugar beets, alfalfa and potentially other crops. Glyphosate is also sprayed on crops to accelerate ripening.

Glyphosate favors the growth of pathogenic bacteria over beneficial bacteria in two ways:

1. Targeting beneficial bacteria which do not have defenses against it

2. Increasing the antibiotic resistance of some pathogenic bacteria

In the first way, glyphosate targets a molecule known as EPSPS. In plants, in many bacteria and in other microbes, a pathway to create amino acids which are necessary for survival relies on the enzyme EPSP synthase (EPSPS). Humans and animals do not have the EPSPS enzyme, so on first glance it would seem that glyphosate would not affect us, even if we ingest it at sub-lethal doses. However, glyphosate potently and specifically targets the EPSPS enzyme in some gut bacteria which do not have defenses against glyphosate. Targeting the enzyme disrupts its functioning.[123,124]

Unfortunately, many beneficial bacteria species such as *Bifidobacterium* and *Lactobacillus* are moderately-to-highly susceptible to the effects of glyphosate.

Additionally and alarmingly, some pathogenic bacteria, such as *Pseudomonas,* can break down glyphosate and use it for an energy source. Also of concern is that harmful bacteria, such as *Salmonella* and *Clostridium* pathogens, are highly resistant to the enzyme-disruption effects of glyphosate.[125] Thus, glyphosate appears to favor the growth of pathogenic bacteria and decrease the growth of helpful gut bacteria.

Glyphosate has been found in the urine, organs and meat of animals. A study in rats showed that at least a third of the administered dose of glyphosate was absorbed from the GI tracts of the rats and it was also found in their bones.[126]

Residues of glyphosate and its breakdown products have been found on GMO soybeans and animal feed and even on non-GMO food.[127] Therefore humans and animals can be exposed to the opportunity to ingest glyphosate.

The second way that glyphosate favors the growth of pathogenic bacteria over beneficial bacteria is that when exposed to glyphosate, some pathogenic bacteria are able to increase their antibiotic resistance.[128] You have already seen that antibiotics take a toll on beneficial bacteria compared to many pathogenic bacteria. Increased antibiotic resistance of pathogenic bacteria due to glyphosate means that regular doses of certain antibiotics will not kill the "bad guys" but will kill the "good guys", and so higher doses will be needed to fight an infection. It may not be clear which dosage of antibiotic is necessary to combat an infection, leading to insufficient treatment of infections.

Glyphosate is also being investigated for interfering with human enzyme systems[129] and is classified by the International Agency for Research on Cancer of the World Health Organization as "probably carcinogenic."[130]

By affecting our gut bacteria, glyphosate affects us. The extent of those effects remains to be determined.

It can be hard to avoid glyphosate completely, but organic foods in the US should have lower levels since glyphosate is not permitted to be used directly on them at the current time.

Disconnect of modern medicine

There is a disconnect of modern medicine to the concept of a whole body. In an effort to 'fix' one part of the body, sometimes another part is harmed. Such is the case, especially with the prescribing of antibiotics, but also of other drugs, without any prescribing of ways to preserve the microbiota balance. As you have seen, many medications can have negative consequences on your gastrointestinal microbiota and more healthcare practitioners have to become aware of this fact and counsel their patients on how to avoid those consequences.

Another example case of a disconnect of modern medicine to the whole body concept is with iron fortification. Iron fortification can be life-saving for people because addressing anemia is one of the first priorities for health. However, indiscriminately adding iron, especially in a non-ideal form, to a person's diet without assessing the state of their GI tract can cause the balance of harmful microbes to probiotic microbes to tip towards the harmful ones. This is because *Bifidobacterium* and *Lactobacillus* only require small amounts of iron for growth depending on the environment they are in, but too much free iron in the intestine from stress, intestinal bleeding, surgery, trauma, iron fortification or dietary supplements can lead to accelerated growth of other, possibly harmful, microbes which flourish in high-iron environments.

This disconnect was demonstrated in a Swiss-led study in Ivory Coast which showed that undesirable fecal *Enterobacteriaceae* (many Gram-negative pathogenic species) increased at the expense of beneficial *Bifidobacterium* and *Lactobacillus* when iron was added to biscuits and given to children who already had an unfavorable ratio of those bacteria.[131]

Any time you are receiving care for any part of your body, it is best to be aware of what that care might be doing to your helpful microorganisms and to take precautionary measures to protect them.

Lack of Adequate Sleep

If you want to lose weight, check your quality of sleep. If you want to fight infections better, check your quality of sleep. If you want to have a healthier microbiota, check your quality of sleep. Basically, if you want to live a healthier life, check your quality of sleep!

You know you need quality sleep, but are you doing things to ensure that you are getting it?

Your sleep-wake cycle is your *circadian rhythm*. Disruption of this circadian rhythm, or clock, is associated with a wide range of diseases including obesity, diabetes, cancer, cardiovascular disease and lowered immunity.

Biological clocks in archaea, bacteria and eukaryota (cells with nuclei, like yours) all are influenced by the daily rhythms of light caused by the earth's rotation.

Your body sleep-wake cycles do not affect only you. Studies have shown, in both mice and humans, that when sleep is disrupted by things like jet lag or a change in shift work, not only do your cells suffer but the cells of some of your microbiota do, too.[132,133] Certain beneficial species, such as *Lactobacillus*, appear to be more affected by disruptions than other species.

The takeaway here is that one of the ways a normal routine in adequate sleep helps you is through your microbiota. So treat your microbiota well by eating real, whole foods. Also, make sleep a bigger priority in your life to take advantage of your outnumbered status and keep dysbiosis in check!

Sleep disruption plays a role in stress, too, which is the next topic.

Stress

All of the topics discussed in this chapter about why you probably do not have enough probiotics ultimately relate to stress on the body. Although we each have our own definitions of what stress means to us, I like the definition that stress can be defined as the brain's response to any demand.[134]

What a lot of events that are typically viewed as stressful have in common is that they involve change of some sort, whether positive or negative, whether brought about suddenly or over a period of time: a change in work status, a change in routine, a change in health, a change in family status, a change in living location, etc. The change can be physical, mental or emotional. Sometimes it is the lack of control of a situation (such as rush-hour traffic) that causes stress.

It is your brain's perception of an event that determines whether or not it will be stressful to you. Some events, like almost hitting a deer while driving during twilight, or witnessing a violent episode, are real and will be stressful to nearly everyone. Other events, like a lunch meeting with the boss, may be real to everyone or may be perceived to be more stressful to some people than to others. Still other stressors, such as an imbalance in gut flora, may not even be noticeable to your conscious mind, yet your brain is sensing a stressor from an immune response.

The brain's response then sets a cascade of reactions in your body into motion that result in increased stress-hormone and stress-chemical levels. These hormones and chemicals, in turn, cause the classic rapid heartbeat, faster breathing, tense muscles, sweating, decrease in digestion, and heightened awareness, among other symptoms, that you experience from an acute stressor.

Stress itself is not always bad. Humans evolved to be able to react to an acute short-term stressor, such as being chased by a beast, by running or fighting (flight or fight). Stressing your muscles and bones during workouts causes them to become stronger. Acute stress during an exam or competition can help you focus. Stress can provide purpose and meaning to life.

When the acute stressor has passed, humans are then supposed to resume their normal levels of stress hormones and chemicals. Unfortunately, in these complicated times with nearly 24-hour access to everything, the acute stressors are not always easily identifiable as one thing (like the charging beast) or they do not go away (like the beast eventually would). The acute stressors turn into chronic stressors that go on and on. When stress exceeds your ability to manage it, be it acute and/or chronic, is when it can cause problems for you.

Stressors of all sorts, whether emotional or psychological (like anger or fear), mental (like when taking exams) and/or physical (such as exercise overtraining, crowding, noise, heat, lack of sleep and foods incompatible with you) can cause the balance of your microbes to be disrupted.

In general, the response to stress results in an increase in non-probiotic microorganisms and usually a decrease of beneficial lactic acid bacteria (*Lactobacillus* and *Bifidobacterium*, in particular) in both humans and animals.[135,136]

Think not only of what this means to you but of what this means for conventionally-raised CAFO (confined animal feeding operations) animals such as chickens, pigs, turkeys and cattle and it is easy to see that their stressors may be one reason why antibiotic use and probiotic use is widespread in those operations.

Stress causes dysbiosis which then causes more stress in a self-perpetuating cycle.

I encourage you to look at all aspects of your life and see where you can decrease your stress before you develop serious health effects from it. Stress is linked to heart disease, asthma development and complications, obesity, diabetes, headaches, accelerated aging, depression and anxiety, among others, and yes, even to disrupted microbiota (dysbiosis) in the GI tract.

Looking Ahead

Probiotics definitely have a place in a plan for health, as the chapter on the benefits of probiotics shows. This chapter just showed you things you may be taking or doing which damage your beneficial microbiota. Take a critical look at everything in your life, but be gentle with yourself. Drastic changes in behavior usually do not happen overnight. Resolve to figure out the causes of why you take what you take and act like you do. Once you are armed with that information, then you can start to make changes for the better, adding things like probiotics into your routine.

Remember that similar to the consensus that you cannot eat a poor diet and expect exercise to keep you healthy, you also cannot eat a poor diet, do no exercise, take medications indiscriminately, stress incessantly, sleep horribly, have other lifestyle habits that are harmful to you and still expect probiotics to correct for all of that and keep you healthy.

Before you continue on your journey to use probiotics to your advantage, it is helpful to know what the adverse effects may be. Those effects are the subject of the next chapter.

CHAPTER 8

Side Effects of Probiotics

There are but a few side effects of probiotics, compared to all of those health benefits listed in Chapter 6. If you know about them in advance, you will save yourself from surprises. After all, when you are trying to establish a favorable gut environment, the last thing you need is to undermine your success by making rookie mistakes.

Unlike medications, which can have benefits but also very long lists of scary side effects, the downside to probiotics is minimal. **If you are generally healthy, the side effects are usually mild:**

- Some of the probiotic microbes produce gases; this is why you must gradually introduce probiotics into your body so that your microbiota can adjust and not cause you discomfort with increased passing of gas.

- Some of the microorganisms can cause an upset in your digestion, such as increased bowel movements. Probiotics will reconfigure your intestinal flora and influence your immune, digestion, nervous and endocrine systems. This is another reason to introduce probiotics gradually.

- Taking probiotics can result in a Herxheimer reaction, which is a reaction to the LPS and other endotoxins released by the death of harmful microbes[137]. This reaction can include headache, fever, chills, foggy thinking, muscle pain, anxiety, and gastrointestinal upset, among others. If the reaction is severe, you may need to reduce the amount you are taking in. Usually the duration is short. If ever in doubt, seek the help of a qualified health professional.

- Some fermented products can have histamine in them; use proper judgment if histamine intake is a problem for you.

- There is the rare possibility that some of the bacteria might carry genes that could possibly transfer antibiotic resistance genes to the host, although most strains used do not have this capability.

- There is also the possibility that some of the bacteria and yeasts can translocate, or leave their original location, and end up causing an infection elsewhere. However, these instances are very rare if a person is generally healthy.

If you have a suppressed immune system, or are under a doctor's care, or have any concerns at all, please check with your doctor before consuming probiotics.

If your doctor approves, **consider using whole, raw food and drink sources of beneficial microbes first** before supplementing with probiotic supplements or probiotic-fortified foods and drinks. Doing so could potentially prevent any rogue infections caused by a leaky gut. Your body will recognize the fermented whole, raw food and drink sources as nutrition. And you'll be saving money by eating nutritious food that has extra benefits.

Again, **introduce probiotic foods, drinks and supplements gradually.** Some of the readers of my PowerOfProbiotics.com website have had severe reactions to probiotics when taking them unsupervised. The state of, and residents in, your GI tract can affect how you react, so tread slowly at first. You should not assume that a probiotic will be safe or effective under all conditions and in all people. It is possible that a certain probiotic, given in different situations, may have a beneficial effect, no effect at all, or an adverse effect.[138] Starting slowly will help you potentially avoid any side effects of probiotics, and soon you'll be reaping the health benefits.

Now that you are cautioned about possible side effects from probiotics, it is time to explore the probiotic microbes.

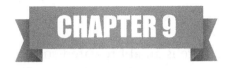

CHAPTER 9

Introduction to the Major Probiotics

There are 5 main probiotics genera (plural of genus) showing the most promise of all bacteria for contributing to health. The main ones to know to use probiotics to your advantage are:

- *Bacillus*
- *Bifidobacterium*
- *Lactobacillus*
- *Saccharomyces*
- *Streptococcus*

Other used genera are *Enterococcus,* and even *Clostridium* and *E. coli*, but these are much less common.

The website, www.powerofprobiotics.com , has more information on each of the 5 main genera and their most significant species and strains. I highly recommend that you visit this very informative site. The growth of the probiotics industry is exploding, and it is much easier and more-timely to update a website than a book.

In the meantime, here is an abbreviated summary of each of the main probiotic genera. I made an analogy for each of them to help you envision what they are like.

Bacillus: The Shapeshifting Transformers of the Probiotics World

Bacillus is a genus of Gram-positive, rod-shaped bacteria in the Firmicutes kingdom that is found widespread in the environment. As a result, **they are often mistakenly called "soil organisms"** or "soil bacteria", although they can be found in soil, water, dust and air. As such, it is no surprise that they were detected in food products such as rice, milk, other grains and vegetables.[139]

This genus is composed of approximately 77 very different species of bacteria ranging from beneficial bacteria like some *Bacillus coagulans* strains to deadly bacteria like *Bacillus anthrax* strains. Most researchers agree that *Bacillus* species do not colonize mucous membranes in the body permanently, so they are transient, and have been recovered in feces in average amounts of 10,000 CFU/g without supplementation.[140,141]

Bacillus is in the same scientific class as *Lactobacillus*, so the two species share some genes including those which allow for the production of lactic acid. As shown in Chapter 6, lactic acid makes the environment too acidic for pathogens to survive.

What makes these microbes unusual in the beneficial bacteria probiotics world are 4 things:[141-145]

1. They act like transforming shapeshifters. These bacteria form endospores (so they are *sporulating*) under stressful conditions. These endospores have tough outer coatings that protect the dormant bacteria inside. This protection can last for years and can be resistant to extreme heat, radiation, extreme freezing, drying, and chemical disinfectants. The spores of some species are stated to be 2 to 8 times more resistant to antibiotics than the vegetative cells. When conditions are favorable for growth, the endospore converts to a vegetative cell which can thrive.

2. Because of the spore-forming ability, *Bacillus* probiotics that are guaranteed to be in spore form may not have to be refrigerated. Always read label directions to be sure.

3. Some *Bacillus* bacteria have whip-like flagella that allow them to be motile (move independently).

4. Most of these spore-forming bacteria thrive best in an oxygenated environment, although some of them can survive in minimal aerobic conditions, like your intestines, too.

To me, a *Bacillus* is similar to a shapeshifting Transformer® in the way it can carry out its intended functions yet be a virtually indestructible entity when things are not going as planned.

Two species of *Bacillus* bacteria have strains that may be classified as probiotics: *Bacillus coagulans* and *Bacillus subtilis*, although there are other species such as *indicus, licheniformis* and *clausii* that are sometimes used. Strain identification is critical with *Bacillus* probiotics.

For more information on *Bacillus*, please see www.powerof-probiotics.com

Bacillus coagulans:

Bacillus coagulans (B. coagulans) is a bacterium found widespread in the environment and used in many industrial applications. Some strains, but not all strains, are used as probiotics and the EFSA (European Food Safety Authority) has this species on its QPS (Qualified Presumption of Safety) list.

Until 1974 it was classified as *Lactobacillus sporogenes* because it produces lactic acid, but it is not considered to be a lactic-acid bacterium (LAB) such as *Lactobacillus, Bifidobacterium, Streptococcus, Lactococcus, Pediococcus,* etc. because it forms endo-spores and the LAB do not.

This ability to form endospores makes the probiotic strains of the species *Bacillus coagulans* attractive for use in numerous food products ranging from breads to frozen yogurts.[146]

The probiotic strains are considered to be probiotics because in their vegetative (growing) state: [143,145,147-150]

1. They produce lactic acid to make conditions unsuitable for pathogenic bacteria.

2. They produce antimicrobial substances.

3. Once inside the body, these strains survive passage through the stomach and begin to transform into active cells in the intestines.

4. Based on animal studies, they are not thought to colonize the intestines on a permanent basis.

5. Based on animal studies, they showed no toxicity.

6. They are suited to the temperature of the body.

7. They produce butyrate (a short-chain fatty acid) to nourish intestinal cells.

8. They do not contain genes that encode known toxins.

9. They stimulate the immune system.

Some strains of *Bacillus coagulans*, such as GBI-30, 6086, have been studied specifically for:

- Rheumatoid arthritis
- Abdominal pain and bloating
- Diarrhea-predominant IBS (irritable bowel syndrome)
- Viral respiratory tract infections

Identification and verification of the strain is extremely important; *Bacillus coagulans* has some strains used in veterinary products which produce toxins that can cause diarrhea.

For more information on the *Bacillus coagulans*, please see www.powerofprobiotics.com

Bacillus subtilis:

Bacillus subtilis is another *Bacillus* species that is found in many environments. Certain strains are used in the production of natto, a traditional Japanese dish of fermented soybeans. It is one of the best-characterized (and possibly most genetically-manipulated) species of all Gram–positive bacteria since its discovery in the 1870's. Like *Bacillus coagulans, B. subtilis* is able to move about due to flagella.[151]

It also is one of those microbes in which the strain used is extremely important because some products have listed "*B. subtilis*" on their labels when in fact they were another *Bacillus* species, such as *Bacillus cereus*, known to produce toxins.

This mislabeling may be because the *B. subtilis* classification has undergone changes over the years. Studies show that there is a high genetic variety in *B. subtilis* even in strains harvested from the same source.[145,152,153]

Some strains are capable of producing toxins. *B. subtilis* in general is known to produce an extracellular toxin and an enzyme which disrupts cell membranes of mammals (and humans are mammals). However, some strains do not possess those factors. *B. subtilis* can cross mucosal barriers and be taken up by immune cells in the GI tract, although no evidence in one study has been found of them reproducing once they crossed the barrier.[154,155]

The toxins produced by some *B. subtilis* are reported to have low disease potential aside from being capable of causing allergic reactions to workers in fermentation facilities. Therefore, *Bacillus subtilis* is thought to have a weak ability to cause disease in humans unless the number of bacteria a person consumes is very high or the immune status of the person is very low.

Also, *Bacillus subtilis* as a whole is able to acquire genetic material from other bacteria, making identification that much more important. Research has shown that over the years as the type strain for this species has been distributed to various laboratories, the strain has become contaminated in some labs. Strict storage and reproductive facilities are required to keep this species genetically pure.[156]

Some other probiotic attributes that *Bacillus subtilis* may have are:[140,142,155-160]

- Is considered to be a normal, albeit very minor, inhabitant of the gut in animals and humans

- Survives passage through the GI tract

- Some strains adhere to human intestinal cells in the laboratory

- Increases immune reaction of intestinal cells which is helpful against pathogens but may not be helpful in auto-immune conditions

- Is able to promote GALT development

- Can persist in the GI tract, increase its numbers and then re-sporulate, if necessary. Whether this is good or is bad remains to be discovered.

- Communicates with intestinal cells to maintain gut barrier function

- Can produce vitamin K2 and B vitamins

For more information on *Bacillus subtilis*, please see www. powerofprobiotics.com

Bifidobacterium: The Security Officers of the Probiotics World

Bifidobacterium are probiotic LAB (lactic-acid bacteria) celebrities. Although you need more than one species of probiotic microbe to be healthy, these probiotic microbes play critical roles in your health.

I think *Bifidobacterium* can be likened to security officers. Just as the mere presence of security officers may prevent people from doing bad things and allows the officers to call for backup in the case of an event, the presence of members of *Bifidobacterium* can keep the peace to discourage pathogens and the production of toxins from foods and other microbes.

They can cause other microbes that live in the intestines to perform helpful duties that they otherwise wouldn't do, and they can communicate with your immune system and other microbes to be either anti-inflammatory or pro-inflammatory, as needed.[161] Like security officers, *Bifidobacterium* are there to protect the premises.

Scientifically, *Bifidobacterium* is a genus of Gram-positive, anaerobic, non-sporulating, non-motile (incapable of moving about on their own due to the lack of flagella), usually branched rod-shaped bacteria in the Actinobacteria kingdom. Many strains have GRAS status in the US and, as a whole, *Bifidobacterium* is well-characterized, non-pathogenic and non-toxigenic.

To date, about 32 different bifido species have been identified, although most of them are very similar in their genetic make-up. Sometimes they are called *bifidobacteria* or *bifido* or even *Bifidobacillus*. Some of the well-known probiotic species you may encounter and that have QPS status by the EFSA are:

- *B. adolescentis*
- *B. animalis*
- *B. bifidum*
- *B. breve*

- *B. infantis*
- *B. lactis*
- *B. longum*

Because they are anaerobic and can't tolerate oxygen-rich environments, you won't find them naturally widespread in food and drink products that are easily exposed to air. In humans, they are found in the gastrointestinal (GI) tract, breast milk and the female vagina and urogenital tract. These good bacteria are some of the first microbes to take up residence in the sterile gastro-intestinal (GI) tract of newborns, and they dominate the intestines in breast-fed babies. As babies age and are weaned, the bifidobacteria numbers and species change as the diet changes.

Typically, their numbers continue to decrease with age.[162] Their total numbers are influenced by diet, lifestyle and overall health. They are found in the highest numbers in the colon (large intestine), although they only amount to 3-6% of the total flora in adult feces. *Bifidobacterium* can be decimated by most common antibiotics.

Bifidobacterium, along with *Lactobacillus*, are also some of the most well-known probiotics and are an important part of your gut flora. Both species produce lactic-acid from carbohydrates to lower the pH to make conditions inhospitable for many pathogenic microbes (and to aid in mineral absorption from food) and make vitamins, bacteriocins (antibacterial chemicals) and antibiotic-like substances. Both have significant health benefits on the digestive and immune systems. In fact, many of the benefits of probiotics listed in Chapter 6 are due to *Bifidobacterium* and *Lactobacillus* species.

Adding to the *Bifidobacterium* arsenal of beneficial effects is the capability to also produce acetic acid, a short-chain fatty acid (SCFA). Acetic acid is more effective at reducing the growth of yeasts and molds than is lactic acid. Acetic acid can also be used as energy by the human body.

Producing both lactic and acetic acids and other beneficial compounds makes *Bifidobacterium* a probiotic qualified to be in the colon, where the opportunity for disease to flourish is greater because fecal transit time slows.[163]

A few other benefits of *Bifidobacterium* are:[162,164-173]

- Many of them establish residence inside us so they can crowd out harmful microbes, prevent them from attaching to our cells and/or displace them if they do attach.

- Maintenance of the intestinal barrier to prevent leaky gut

- The production of ethanol which may be protective to us against naturally-occurring methanol from foods

- The production of small amounts of formic acid which may be antibacterial against pathogenic microbes

- The production of antimicrobial and antibiotic substances in some species

- The ability of many species to withstand stomach acid for short time periods and survive in bile acids

- The ability to breakdown any proteins that reach your colon without being digested, so that contents in your colon don't putrefy and become nasty

- Help with lactose intolerance

- The production of some B vitamins by some species

- The ability to prevent or help constipation problems or IBS by helping your colon function normally

- Some species may be helpful for allergies, lowering of cholesterol, antibiotic-associated diarrhea, and gastrointestinal upset with rumbling bowels, gas, constipation and diarrhea.

- Most, but not all, species have an anti-inflammatory effect.

For more information on *Bifidobacterium*, please visit www.powerofprobiotics.com.

Lactobacillus: The Police of the Probiotics World

Lactobacillus are LAB (lactic-acid bacteria) superstar probiotics, next in line after *Bifidobacterium.* Together, both of these species of good bacteria work to help you be healthy.

As previously stated, *Lactobacillus* and *Bifidobacterium* are some of the most well-known probiotics and are an important, albeit small, percentage of your gut flora. *Lactobacillus* and *Bifidobacterium* share a few common genes. Both species produce lactic-acid from carbohydrates to lower the pH to make conditions inhospitable for many pathogenic microbes (and to aid in mineral absorption from food) and make vitamins, bacteriocins (antibacterial chemicals) and antibiotic-like substances. Both have significant health benefits on the digestive and immune systems. In fact, many of the benefits of probiotics listed in Chapter 6 are due to *Bifidobacterium* and *Lactobacillus* species.

While *Bifidobacterium* may be more like security guards in keeping us healthy, *Lactobacillus* to me are more like the police because their actions are more targeted. In general, like the bifidos,

Lactobacillus bacteria:

- Can keep the peace by their presence
- Some can cause other microbes that live in the intestines to perform helpful duties that they otherwise wouldn't do
- Communicate with your cells and with other microbes

Additionally, *Lactobacillus* can also mount massive attacks against harmful microbes all along your GI tract. In contrast, most bifidos are found in the colon.

Scientifically, *Lactobacillus* is a genus of Gram-positive, nonsporulating, and non-motile (incapable of moving about on their own due to the lack of flagella), rod-shaped bacteria in the Firmicutes kingdom. Most of them are able to survive in small amounts of oxygen. Unlike *Bifidobacterium, Lactobacillus* is a diverse genetic genus with the different species having different capabilities.

These good bacteria have GRAS (generally recognized as safe) status in the US, meaning that there is general recognition of their safety through experience based on common use in foods. Although some of the species may be associated with dental caries or with infections in immune-system compromised people, most of the time they are beneficial bacteria.

These microbes are commonly found in the environment. For instance, *Lactobacillus* microbes are found in everyday fermented/cultured foods and drinks such as yogurt, kefir, sauerkraut, miso, cheese, kombucha and many others.

In humans, they are found in the gastrointestinal (GI) tract, from the mouth, the nasal passages (sinuses), the throat, the esophagus, the stomach, the small intestine (the duodenum, jejunum and ileum sections) and the colon (large intestine). *Lactobacillus* are the most popular genus in the last section of the small intestine, the ileum. Once established, they tend to remain life-long under normal circumstances and with consistent replacement. They are also found in the female vagina and urogenital tract. Similar to *Bifidobacterium,* the total numbers of *Lactobacillus* bacteria in your body are influenced by diet, lifestyle and general health.

Many, but not all, species of these bacteria are able to withstand stomach acid and bile acids and are able to attach to the cells lining the GI tract and interact with them.

Additional benefits of *Lactobacillus* are:[174-184]

- Many of them establish residence inside us so they can crowd out harmful microbes, prevent them from attaching to our cells and/or displace them if they do attach.

- Maintenance of the intestinal barrier to prevent leaky gut

- *Lactobacillus* prefer different kinds of carbohydrates depending on their species. Some of them can use lactose, which is nice to know if you have lactose intolerance.

- For those that do not colonize inside us, ingesting them can cause temporary increases in numbers in your body and temporary benefits.

- Some of them produce vitamins.

- Some of them produce short-chain fatty acids.

- Some of them produce hydrogen peroxide which kills pathogens.

- Most produce bacteriocins (antibacterials) and antibiotic chemicals, depending on their living conditions.
- Species can induce either a strong or weak pro-inflammatory response, and an anti-inflammatory response, depending on the perceived need.

Common species you may encounter and that have QPS status by the EFSA are:

- *L. acidophilus*
- *L. brevis*
- *L. bulgaricus*
- *L. casei*
- *L. fermentum*
- *L. gasseri*
- *L. helveticus*
- *L. johnsonii*
- *L. paracasei*
- *L. plantarum*
- *L. reuteri*
- *L. rhamnosus*
- *L. salivarius.*

Since there are so many species in this genus, you'll have to learn more about each of them individually to know the differences in what they can do. For more information on *Lactobacillus*, please see www.powerofprobiotics.com .

Saccharomyces: The Special Forces of the Probiotics World

Saccharomyces is unique in the probiotics world because it is a yeast. As a yeast, it is not affected by stomach acid, bile and antibiotics so it is able to survive harsh conditions which might kill other probiotic species. However, anti-fungal medications can kill it.

I think *Saccharomyces* can be considered the Special Forces of the probiotics world because it goes in, does its job very well and then leaves.

The main species used as a probiotic is *S. boulardii.* Unlike invasive *Candida* species of yeasts, *S. boulardii* is unable to penetrate into tissues nor colonize the GI tract, so it performs its beneficial functions as a passer-by.

It's not a yeast to be afraid of, **unless you're allergic to yeast**, of course. Precautions have to be taken if you have any type of catheter, port or IV, or are immune-compromised, but if that situation applies to you, then please check with your doctor before using *any* probiotics.

Some of the probiotic functions of *S. boulardii* include:[185-194]

- Stimulated immunity in response to pathogens
- Ability to help with lactose intolerance
- Prevention of traveler's diarrhea
- Prevention and treatment of antibiotic-associated diarrhea
- Prevention of intestinal infections by pathogens such as *C. difficile, E. coli* and *C. albicans*

- Prevention of translocation (re-location to another organ) of *Candida albicans* from the GI tract to other organs

- Reduction of the virulence of many gut pathogens, including parasites

- Potential to injure *H. pylori*, making it useful when added to an antibiotic regimen

- Potential to improve outcomes in ulcerative colitis and Crohn's disease therapies

- Potential to prevent reactions to food antigens in very young infants who have compromised intestines

- For more information on *Saccharomyces*, please visit www.powerofprobiotics.com.

Streptococcus: Two Good Apples in the Bunch

The name *Streptococcus* can raise fear in people and with good reason (think about strep throat, meningitis and bacterial pneumonia, to name a few). While some streptococci are highly pathogenic, most of them live harmlessly inside us.

However, there are two good apples in the bunch, *Streptococcus thermophilus* and *Streptococcus salivarius,* which are probiotics.

Scientifically, *Streptococcus* is a genus of Gram-positive, non-sporulating, and non-motile (incapable of moving about on their own due to the lack of flagella), spherical-shaped, chain-forming, lactic-acid bacteria in the Firmicutes kingdom.

S. thermophilus

S. thermophilus is in the European Qualified Presumption of Safety list of food bacteria and is a generally recognized as a safe species (GRAS status). It has a long documented history of safe use in food and its genome is devoid of potential virulence functional genes. It is one of the bacteria that make yogurt, well, yogurt.

In addition to its contribution to yogurt-making, *S thermophilus* also is a probiotic that has many benefits. For example, many strains:[195-202]

- Are used in the manufacture of some cheeses such as Swiss, Limburger and Brick
- Can survive passage to the intestines
- Can help maintain gut integrity to prevent a leaky gut
- Enhance lactose digestion
- Can help compete with pathogenic microbes
- May produce bacteriocins
- May help with gastritis by modulating the immune response and increasing the thickness of the protective gastric layer of mucus.
- May produce folate, a B vitamin

S. salivarius

Streptococcus salivarius, as you might expect from the name, is often found in the saliva. It is closely related to *S. thermophilus*. It can be found throughout the GI tract, but is predominantly colonized in the mouth and back of the throat.[203]

Here are a few of the benefits that some strains of *S. salivarius* provide:[204-207]

- Inhibit pathogenic strains of *Streptococcus*
- Antagonize the pathogens involved in bad breath, tooth decay, gum disease and sore throat by preventing their adhesion to cells and their abilities to form biofilms and/or by directly killing them with antibiotic compounds
- Secrete antimicrobials
- Are anti-inflammatory
- Proved to be protective in a mouse model of colitis
- One strain is classified as a food in Australia and New Zealand.
- *Streptococcus salivarius* are common in the mouth and make up to 40% of all the bacteria in the normal healthy mouth. Some strains can provide oral health benefits when taken regularly.

For more information on *Streptococcus*, please visit www.powerofprobiotics.com.

Onward

In this chapter, you read about the 5 major genera of probiotics and hopefully the analogies will help you to more easily remember them. You also may have looked for more details about some of them from the PowerOfProbiotics.com website. In the next chapter, you will see where you can find probiotics and when to take them to use them to your advantage.

CHAPTER 10

Where to Get Probiotics and When to Take Them?

You learned a lot about probiotics at this point, from the basics of

- What they are
- Who benefits from them
- How they are named, and
- Where they live

To more advanced information about

- How they work
- How they benefit your health
- Why you are probably lacking in them
- How to get started with them and what side effects may occur, and
- Who the major players are and what their actions may be.

Now it is important to understand where to get probiotics and beneficial microbes and when to take them so that you are advantageously using sources and timing to your benefit.

As explained before, beneficial bacteria and yeasts had been consumed by the human race for generations, yet the modern diet is *sadly* lacking in them. Approximately 25% of people consuming a Western-style diet have absolutely NO *Lactobacillus* in their feces. That means that twenty-five percent of people eating Western-diet foodstuff, devoid of real nutrition, do not have the benefits given by *Lactobacillus*. Are you one of them?

One of the easiest ways to increase beneficial microbes, some of which may have probiotic actions but do not fit the exact definition of probiotics, in your gut is to eat raw, fresh produce. Raw, whole foods are foods that look like they were just picked off the tree, vine or plant stem, or dug up as a root of a plant such as those you would find in vegetable and fruit gardens, at a farmer's market stand, or in the fresh produce section of your grocery store or supermarket.

Whole foods have the complete nutrients of the food. For example, an apple has fiber, vitamins, minerals and phytonutrients (plant compounds). Whole foods are excellent sources of prebiotics to feed the probiotics, too. An apple is a whole food. Apple juice is not a whole food. It is basically sugar water with vitamins added back into it by manufacturers.

Brown rice is a whole food. White rice is not. Steel-cut oats is a whole food. Ready-to-eat cereals are not. Raw cacao is a whole food. Milk chocolate is not.

Raw, fresh produce has microbes, such as *Lactobacillus planta-rum*, on it and if you eat organically, washing thoroughly with water is usually enough to remove dirt and potentially harmful microbes. So, for example, coleslaw (go easy on the sweetener!) is more microbe-friendly than sautéed cabbage and carrots, even though both contain the amazing vegetable, cabbage.

Another easy way to increase beneficial microbes is to consume fermented food and drink products. Fermentation preserves food from spoilage and allows beneficial microbes on raw food (or in an added culture) to flourish. *Sorry*, wine, beer and other alcoholic drinks are fermented to the point of having too much alcohol in them to be healthy sources of beneficial microbes.

From the above example of coleslaw, instead of mixing the cabbage, carrots and herbs with a sauce to make coleslaw, taking the ingredients and submerging them in salt water will yield sauerkraut in a matter of days, thanks to the fermenting actions of the bacteria on the cabbage. Sauerkraut and coleslaw are both packed with nutrients, but the sauerkraut has several advantages including increased populations of beneficial bacteria, fewer populations of harmful bacteria, little to no sugar, easier digestibility and higher levels of vitamins C, B and possibly K. Chapter 13 has several recipes utilizing cabbage.

The tanginess of the sauerkraut is caused partially by lactic acid secreted by the beneficial microbes. For a video and directions on how to do make sauerkraut in bulk, see www.powerofprobiotics/ Sauerkraut.html . Be sure to eat raw sauerkraut and not heat-killed jarred or canned varieties.

Many different types of foods, beyond sauerkraut and the familiar yogurt, can be fermented to yield microbial benefits. Kefir, kimchi, kombucha, kvass, pickles (not the ones in vinegar), gingerbeer, some cheeses, some sausages, raw honey, miso, natto, some olives, raw cacao, tempeh, raw milk and raw buttermilk are just some of the foods and drinks in the Westernized world that contain beneficial microbes to help you gain control over the potentially harmful microbes. I included some recipes for using fermented foods and drinks in Chapter 13. You can also attend a workshop on fermentation if you need someone to guide you step-by-step.

What if you don't like the taste of fermented foods and drinks? As you learned in Chapter 7, modern-day processed food is laced with chemicals to make you like the food and even crave it. Fermented foods and drinks have tastes and textures that are very different from those in processed foods. Don't worry, however. All you need to do is keep an open mind and start with a tiny amount of a fermented food or drink. You may dislike the taste or smell of something at first, but you can learn to adapt to it over time. For most people, including children, learning to tolerate, and even like, different tastes and textures is completely possible with small, repeated exposures. Research shows that it can take 10 to 16 repeated exposures before acceptance to a new food occurs. For people with diagnosed sensory sensitivities, this can be more of a challenge, but is still doable. Don't give up trying too quickly!

Just remember that you do not have to LOVE the taste of a fermented food or drink. Appreciating how good it is for you can help you get over the mental hurdle. Pairing the fermented food or drink with something else can enhance the flavors of both, as you will see in Chapter 13.

Sometimes a good way to get beneficial microbes is to consume products that are fortified with them. *Bacillus* species are one example of this as they can be added to frozen foods, room-temperature foods and hot foods and still survive. *Lactobacillus* and *Bifidobacterium* can be added to cool foods as long as their favorable environmental conditions are met. *Streptococcus thermophilus* multiplies fastest at 95-108 degrees F and that is why milks are heated and kept warm when making yogurt. Refrigeration slows down the fermentation process.

There are four excellent reasons for including fermented or probiotic-fortified foods in your diet. The first reason is the real beauty of eating and/or drinking food or beverages with beneficial microbes: you are nourishing your body with the kinds of sustenance that it is accustomed to having for overall health. You will be getting all the vitamins, minerals, healthy fats and plant compounds from them that your body needs for optimal health, plus the benefits of the helpful microbes. And all of this will happen naturally any time you feed your hunger or thirst.

Another beautiful thing about incorporating sources of beneficial microbes into your routine is that it is always helpful to consistently take in those microbes. Since some microbes are transient, meaning that they pass through, you have to keep ingesting them to keep reaping their benefits.

A third bonus from eating and/or drinking sources of beneficial microbes is that you will inoculate your digestive tract, starting in the mouth, through the esophagus and in the stomach, not simply in the intestines as you would with a swallowed supplement.

The last excellent reason for eating and/or drinking most food or beverage sources of beneficial microbes is that you get the beneficial supernatant with them. The *supernatant* is the medium on which the microbes grow and release some of their health-giving substances. While probiotics research focuses on the particular microbes, other research shows that the supernatant has healthy properties, even without the microbes present.

If, however, there is any doubt about how many beneficial microbes, including probiotics, you are consuming, you can always take a probiotic supplement. Doing so can be especially helpful for one of the many conditions that probiotics have been shown to benefit and for basic health maintenance. Additionally, probiotic supplements can be taken in acute situations to provide a blitzkrieg to overwhelm the pathogenic microbes.

It is best to take most probiotic supplements, especially the LAB (lactic-acid bacteria), with at least some food so the food can provide nutrients for the microbes and also can buffer the acid in your stomach. Sometimes an empty stomach can have a pH of less than 2 which can:

- Make it harder for probiotics to survive
- Make you feel nauseous if you put supplements in your empty stomach

Do not take probiotics with hot liquids, nor sprinkle them on hot foods, as the heat can damage all but designated *Bacillus* probiotics. Likewise, do not subject foods and drinks with beneficial microbes in them to heat unless the packaging says so.

Do not take probiotics (with the exception of *Saccharomyces boulardii*) within 3 hours of taking antibiotics or herbals with antibiotic properties because the antibiotic substances may kill the probiotics.

Of course, if there is ever any question about whether any of these options for sources of probiotics and other beneficial microbes are right for you, it is recommended that you consult with a qualified healthcare professional.

Probiotic supplements are big business these days and how to choose them is the topic of the next chapter.

CHAPTER 11

How to Choose a Source of Purchased Probiotics, Including a Probiotic Supplement

As seen in the last chapter, probiotics and other beneficial microbes are available in a wide variety of foods, drinks and supplements. Additionally, prebiotics are naturally found in a variety of whole foods.

Many times people want to buy sources of probiotics and beneficial microbes, instead of trying to make them, or they need extra help from specific microbes that are known to be in purchased products. How do you know which products to choose? It is easy to feel overwhelmed when sifting through the different products on the market. The information below will help to guide you.

Additionally, my website, PowerOfProbiotics.com, has many reviews of different purchased products and those reviews detail many of the considerations listed below. New reviews are added regularly.

There are 14 considerations when deciding which sources of probiotics from purchased products will give you an advantage:

1. Your condition: Where is the problem and what is your current state? What medications are you currently using?

2. Your expectations: What is your goal?

3. Your sensitivities, intolerances and allergies: Do you have any restrictions on what you can take?

4. The need for prebiotics

5. The types of probiotics: Where do the probiotics act and what are the substances produced by and actions of the probiotics you are considering?

6. The need for enteric coatings

7. CFU of the food, drink or product: How strong is it?

8. CFU of each probiotic strain: Do the CFU amounts of your desired probiotic strains equal the amounts shown effective in studies?

9. Storage conditions: Are you able to store it properly?

10. Size and dosage recommendations of the product. What is the serving size? Are you able to take the product as recommended?

11. Knowledge of the company

12. Third-party or in-house certification: Are the contents equal to what is listed on the label?

13. Your uniqueness

14. Proprietary formulas

First, you need to consider your body. What are your needs? Do you need security guards, police, shapeshifters and/or transient microbes? For example, where in the body is the focus of your concern?

Are you generally healthy except for this problem or are you dealing with multiple concerns? If you are generally healthy then you may think that you don't need probiotics and other beneficial microbes, and you would be wrong. Good health is not a guaranteed, continuous state; it requires daily maintenance. Just because you may be at your optimal weight does not mean you can neglect exercising. Just because you may have money in your wallet for today's lunch does not mean that you can stop working. Prevention of bad health- and wellbeing-outcomes is not a one-time dosage of something but rather involves the incorporation of preventive measures into your daily life.

If you are generally healthy, the effects from adding sources of probiotics may not be as dramatic as if you were sick, and instead may be subtle. However, that does NOT mean that you are not benefitting from them. Recall from Chapter 7 that you experience many assaults on your digestive tract and its microbiota from things you encounter every day. Replenishing the beneficial microbes keeps the microbiota balanced. One of the best uses of probiotics is in prevention of illness through influences on your digestive, immune, nervous and endocrine systems. It is worth repeating that prevention of illness is easier to achieve than management of an established illness.

If you have multiple concerns, then the place to start is in healing your digestive tract. Probiotics are a critical piece of the gut-healing protocol for re-inoculation with beneficial microorganisms, although they are not the only piece. You may require help from a professional in restoring health to your GI tract. From there, you can target your specific conditions with specific probiotics.

Are you strong enough to handle probiotics? If there is ever any doubt, please consult with a qualified medical professional first.

What medications are you using? What effects might those medications have on your microbiota based on the information in Chapter 7? Are there other options? Always speak to your doctor before discontinuing any prescribed medications.

Second, what are your expectations? Are you expecting miracles for your problems or will you be happy with minor improvement? Are you hoping that your need for medications or surgery will decrease? Are you willing to complement the usage of probiotics with other diet and lifestyle improvements? While probiotics can be life-saving and can have drastic effects on the body, many other times the results are more subtle and take time to show any recognizable signs of improvement. As you saw in Chapter 6, benefits of probiotics are so amazing and widespread, but remember that probiotics, unless classified as a drug, are not meant to treat or cure any disease.

Third, do you have allergies or intolerances to yeasts or histamine that may affect which microbes you can take? Do you have allergies, sensitivities or intolerances to any of the other ingredients in the products? Sometimes the medium on which the microbes were cultured is included with the products. In the past, many probiotics were cultured on a dairy base so traces of milk proteins or lactose were common. Nowadays you can find probiotics that are cultured on non-dairy bases, but some may have traces of soy, or corn maltodextrin (usually as GMO) as a filler, or sugar as a sweetener, or gelatin capsules, for example.

You must read ingredient labels carefully if you have any allergies, sensitivities or intolerances. Look for a product with the least amount of additives. My website highlights possible allergens in products.

Fourth, do you want prebiotics in the formula with the probiotics, also known as synbiotics? Prebiotics are substances which increase the growth of the probiotics. FOS (fructooligosaccharides) and inulin are common ones. Prebiotics + probiotics = synbiotic. Sometimes a prebiotic fiber by itself has beneficial actions on the microbiota, but remember, the right microbes have to be present in the first place in order for them to feast on prebiotics.

Synbiotics are fine if you do not react to the prebiotic fibers. For instance, some people, especially those with IBS, may react badly to the FOS prebiotic. If you take any probiotic supplement with real, whole foods (as I recommend), then the supplement's prebiotic may be inconsequential in comparison to the prebiotics in the foods. Many studies have shown that prebiotic amounts measured in grams, not milligrams, are necessary to have a significant GI effect, yet synbiotics typically contain 100-200 milligrams of a prebiotic. A varied whole foods diet will naturally give you prebiotics.

Fifth, consider the microbes you want or need. Where do they normally live? What substances do they produce? What actions do they have in the body? Is the supernatant part of their healing abilities? The best thing to do when taking anything with probiotics in it, if possible, is to choose the particular strain that has been proven effective for a given condition, if you need help with that condition. As previously mentioned, my website is a great resource for this information.

The **sixth** decision to make is the need for enteric coatings. Enteric coatings are used on many supplements and medications to keep the substance inside protected from stomach and bile acids and to deliver the substance to the targeted site in the digestive tract.

Many enteric coatings, such as oils and algae extracts, are relatively harmless unless you have an allergy to them. However, the potential for the use of dangerous phthalates exists. Phthalates are a group of chemicals commonly used to make plastics more flexible. They are known to be endocrine disruptors, meaning that they have actions in the body which interfere with normally functioning of hormones. Endocrine disruptors are associated with obesity and diabetes, female reproduction problems, male reproduction problems, hormone-sensitive cancers in females, prostate cancer, thyroid problems and others. Phthalates are lesser-known than BPA (bisphenol A), but both have these endocrine-disrupting actions.

Avoid any product that has the word "phthalate" in it, and be suspicious of enteric coatings and/or time-release products. Contact the manufacturer if you have any concerns.

The **seventh** consideration in the choice of a source of purchased probiotics is the strength of the source. How do you know if your product has enough of the desirable microbes? One thing to compare is the CFU.

CFU is an acronym (type of abbreviation) commonly seen on products containing probiotics. It stands for *colony forming unit* and is a measurement of some of the good bacteria and yeasts inside. A colony forming unit is a single bacterium or yeast, or group of bacteria or yeasts, which is/are capable of living and reproducing to form a group of the same bacteria or yeasts. Sometimes products will say "viable cells" which may or may not be exactly equal to CFU.

Microbiologists use CFU to describe the number of active, live organisms instead of the number of all the organisms - dead, inactive and alive - in a laboratory sample. Only the viable organisms are considered to be probiotics. *Viable* means that the microbes are capable of living under the proper circumstances.

You may also see it listed as CFUs - colony forming units. Most probiotic supplements in capsule or tablet form will state the number of colony forming units in the capsule or tablet. Or, if more than one capsule or tablet is the recommended serving size, then the colony forming units listed may be the total in the serving size. The only way to know for sure is to read the package.

Unless individually packaged, most powder probiotic supplements will have a recommended serving size listed and then the colony forming units in that serving size. For example, 1/4 teaspoon may contain 100 billion CFU. Taking a consistent amount of a powder may be difficult, especially if you only want to take one-sixteenth of a teaspoon for 25 billion CFU.

Another way the information may be presented is CFU/g or /ml, meaning colony forming unit per unit of measure, or how many capable-of-living microbes are in a certain measurement. In these cases, you must look at the serving size in g (grams for a solid) or ml (milliliters for a liquid) and perform a mathematics equation.

Multiply the colony forming units per gram or per milliliter by the number of grams or milliliters in the serving size to get the total number of colony forming units.

It is easier to compare products when the standard of measurement is the same, and that's where colony forming units make an "apples to apples" comparison easier. Products that simply state total numbers of good bacteria or yeasts by weight (such as grams) of microbes in a product are not easily compared to other products, and they may not contain enough cultures to make them therapeutic. A total number of grams of probiotics really doesn't mean anything.

Reputable companies should state the number of colony forming units or viable cells and state if the CFU is at the time of manufacture or at product expiration. I believe that it is better if the CFUs stated on the label are at the time of product expiration, not at the time the product was manufactured for several reasons listed below in the storage requirements discussion. This information is very important because it tells you if you really are getting the number of microbes listed on the label when you consume the product.

You see, very few product manufacturers who sell probiotic products actually grow their own microbes. Only certain companies sell the bacteria and yeasts, usually in a raw material form. They either package it themselves or ship it to many product manufacturers who package the raw material in their products, and those are the products you buy and the labels you read.

If a product manufacturer does not have the material tested for the number of colony forming units prior to and after putting it in their packages, the number on the label could be the number that was in the raw material, not the number that is actually in the product you're buying.

The **eighth** consideration in choosing a source of purchased probiotics is the CFU of each strain in the product. Each strain should be present in an amount at least equal to the amount shown in studies to be efficacious for the health condition you have. For instance, if studies show that 10 billion CFU of *L. acidophilus* LA-1 helped a certain condition, then 2 billion CFU in a product cannot be assumed to have the same effect as the 10 billion used in the study. How can you know how many CFU are shown to be beneficial in studies? Check out my website, PowerOfProbiotics.com and subscribe to my newsletter. I share the detailed results of studies with my readers and subscribers.

Relating to the strength of the product, the **ninth** consideration in your choice of which probiotic source to buy is the storage requirements. Do you travel frequently or travel to places where maintaining refrigeration is not possible? Many probiotic foods, drinks and supplements must be refrigerated or the microbes will die. In some cases, probiotic supplements may say that they are *shelf stable*. Shelf stable does not mean that you can subject the probiotics to high heat and humidity, but it means that they can withstand room-temperature conditions. Unless a probiotic label says NOT to refrigerate it, always refrigerate probiotics to preserve their numbers.

There are several ways the colony forming unit listed on the label can decrease so that it is less than that by the time you buy the product. For example, if the original raw material microbe product from the raw material supplier of the microbes was made with a certain number of viable bacteria in it, those bacteria can die if:

- The product wasn't shipped in cool, low-humidity conditions from the raw material supplier to the product manufacturer

- The product manufacturer didn't store the raw material in cool, low-humidity conditions in their warehouse

- The product manufacturer didn't package the raw material in a facility where the temperature and humidity were tightly controlled

- The packaged product wasn't stored in cool, low-humidity conditions in the manufacturer's warehouse

- The packaged product wasn't shipped in cool, low-humidity conditions

- The store (either online or brick-and-mortar) didn't keep the packaged product at low temperature and humidity before you bought it

- You took the product home and left it at room temperature instead of refrigerating it, if that is what the label instructions said to do. Or worse yet, you forgot about it and left it in your hot car.

Some probiotics, such as some freeze-dried *Saccharomyces boulardii* yeast ones, may state on the label NOT to refrigerate it. However, this is rare. **Always read and follow product label instructions and contact the manufacturer if you have any concerns.**

If you use probiotic products from a reputable manufacturer who follows strict handling procedures, you buy your products from a seller who knows how to store the products properly, and you yourself store the product correctly and consume it by the expiration date, the CFU you consume should be at least the amount you were promised.

What if the CFU is not listed? Many times you will only see the words "live cultures", not "probiotics" on purchased products. This is because the numbers of probiotic microbes in them are not high enough to satisfy the World Health Organization's definition of probiotics or the microbes are not technically probiotic microbes.

The National Yogurt Association allows a Live and Active Cultures Seal on yogurts that contain the two probiotics that define yogurt, *Lactobacillus bulgaricus* and *Streptococcus thermophilus*. Other microbes may be added to the yogurt, but those two are required. This seal still does not tell you how many microbes you are consuming because restrictions state that the product must start with 100 million total CFU at time of manufacture.

It is true that products that say "live cultures" on the label may or may not contain enough beneficial microorganisms to be statistically significant in scientific studies. It is also true that sometimes saying "live cultures" is a marketing strategy to lure you into buying a product. So buyer-beware: you may not be getting a significant amount of beneficial microbes and may instead be getting a lot of added sugars and other junk.

The **tenth** consideration when you are considering a bought probiotic deals with serving size. The size of a capsule or tablet can be too big and be a choking hazard for some people. Some probiotic capsules can be opened and mixed in cool drinks or food; others must be kept in the capsule. Some brands, especially for children, are meant to be mixed in water and drunk. Having a source of extra water and a cup in some circumstances, such as on a camping trip, can make taking the supplement difficult. Also, at times, a serving size is only one capsule or tablet, but in other cases, a serving size is 2 or more. You must read the label to know how much you need to take.

The **eleventh** point to ponder during your choice of probiotics is the knowledge of the company selling the product. Some brands of probiotics are sold by people with no knowledge of the characteristics of the microbes they sell. Bigger supplement companies usually, but not always, have the resources to study and carefully choose the microorganisms they include in their products. Some smaller companies (but not all of them, of course) are run by people with more marketing knowledge than scientific background and they contract with the microbe manufacturers to include random or trendy microbes in their products.

Do your research. Find out how the company selling the product is qualified to be doing so.

The **twelfth** consideration is a very important one: good manufacturing practices or third-party certification. Third-party testing means that someone who has no financial interest in the product evaluates the product for three standards:

1. The genetic identity of the microbes inside
2. The numbers of viable microbes in it, and
3. Contamination with toxins or pathogens.

I believe that testing of any probiotic product is crucial for safety and effectiveness, and for companies that cannot do in-house testing, third-party certification is a must. A company that tests the final product for quality assurance is probably a reputable company.

The **thirteenth** consideration when purchasing a source of probiotics is a probably the most important one: to remember your uniqueness. Based on the findings from culture-independent methods discussed in Chapter 4, it is not possible to say that a certain microbe will definitely benefit everyone in every circumstance. Your microbiota and microbiomes are unique to you.

Articles in newspapers and on news sites, while beneficial to some people, may not be relevant to you or help you in your buying decisions. Sometimes the only way to know what works for you at this point in time is by reading about what the research has shown on the PowerOfProbiotics.com website and then trying similar products and diet interventions through trial and error, or by consulting with a qualified professional.

Recall from previous chapters that what seems to be important in health is that the beneficial microbes keep the body balanced. Although the numbers and even species of microbes can vary from healthy person to healthy person, the beneficial FUNCTIONS the microbiome as a whole performs are what matter. For instance, there isn't just one microbe capable of digesting lactose (milk sugar) for you. So if you have Microbe A that does it, and I have Microbe B that does it, our microbes are different but the benefits they provide to us are the same.

You can get the most benefits from probiotics by understanding your condition, your expectations and goals, your sensitivities, your allergies and intolerances, the basics about the probiotics you are considering, the CFU required for your certain condition, the required storage conditions of the product, the serving size and dosage requirements, the qualifications of the producer, the validity of claims made on the label, and what seems to help or hurt your body. My website, www.PowerOfProbiotics.com, is helpful for understanding much of this information.

Additionally, taking in a variety of probiotics from a variety of sources may be the best way to keep your flora diverse and healthy because as you saw in previous chapters, different microbes prefer different environments. Again, check the website for information and for nutritional help in narrowing down the best strains for your needs.

If you are consistently eating or drinking raw, fermented foodstuffs, especially if you make them yourself and incubate them with added probiotic cultures, then you may be consuming enough to be considered "adequate amounts", even if it is not officially declared to be so.

The **fourteenth** and last subtopic in this topic of how to choose a source of purchased probiotics, including a probiotic supplement, is the idea of proprietary formulas. If you think back on the information in this book, I have stressed the importance of knowing the strain of the probiotic(s) you are considering if you are looking for a certain health benefit. Most people are looking for something to help them with a specific condition and so specific strains are desired. Many probiotic products, especially supplements, will only say that the different species listed are blended together in a proprietary formula consisting of a certain number of total CFU or viable cells. Some products will go so far as to even list the other ingredients as general ingredients, such as "vegetable fiber".

Unfortunately for us consumers, many manufacturers are claiming that their probiotic formulas are proprietary and they won't disclose which strains are in the different species. Unless that particular product was used in specific research, you have no idea of what specific conditions it can benefit and in most cases, the label will say that it supports GI and immune health, or something along those vague, structure/function lines. This doesn't automatically mean that the product is inferior to others in any way, it only means that it makes it more difficult to find the exact strain that you may seek for a particular condition and you may have to trust that the reputable manufacturer has the correct strains in it. Other manufacturers use strains that are patented and marketed around the globe and they disclose that information.

If this kind of labeling frustrates you, you are not alone. I completely share your frustration. Manufacturers are trying to comply with general structure/function allowances by governmental regulatory bodies while also getting ahead of their competition by formulating the best mix (in their opinion) of microbes. However, I believe that we consumers need to know what is in our supplements, just like we need to know what is in our food.

Since most probiotic products can only list structure/function claims such as "improves digestion", such broad claims do not help us if we are seeking targeted strains for our particular circumstance. Perhaps, sometime in the future, as companies satisfy the requirements of governmental regulatory bodies and are awarded with stating specific health claims on their products, we consumers will have an easier time choosing the best probiotic supplement for our unique circumstances. Of course, probiotic supplements must be available to the general public and not prescription-only products for that to happen.

When you are faced with the incredible magnitude of information on probiotics on the internet and through the media, it is no wonder that you may feel overwhelmed and not know what to believe. It is not your fault! Review these fourteen points when considering a probiotics product and you will be able to choose those which give you an advantage.

CHAPTER 12

The Magic Bullet?

My goals in writing this book were twofold: one, to dispel many of the misconceptions people have about probiotics; and two, to help you gain an understanding of probiotics so you can use them to your advantage to optimize your health.

In this book, you have learned so much about probiotics, from the basics to more advanced information, in order to fulfill those goals. You began by learning about the 3 main themes that are emerging from international research on the gut microbiota and microbiome:

1. The human gut microbiota and the microbial genome (microbiome) play diverse physiological roles that influence our health and wellbeing.

2. Particularly in the digestive tract, the less diverse the microbial community (and especially with harmful or opportunistic organisms dominating the flora), the less healthy the body can be.

3. Prevention of illness is easier than reaction to established illness.

You now understand how probiotics address those themes based on the details of what you learned in this book:

- Probiotics are, "Live organisms which, when administered in adequate amounts, confer a health benefit on the host".

- Any untampered living thing in the Animal Kingdom has microbes in it; some have beneficial properties and some are probiotics.

- Probiotics and other microbes are named to reflect their genetic lineage. Probiotics should be defined at least at the genus and species levels for general claims and at the strain levels for specific health claims.

- Probiotics and other microbes live in and on our bodies, primarily in major mucosal surfaces. They are very similar to human society in terms of contributions, variety, interactions, clustering and transience. As in any successful society, the contributions of those that benefit the society must outweigh the negative influences of others. Probiotics may be small percentages of the total microbial numbers, but their benefits are critical to health.

- Probiotics work by primarily influencing you digestive, immune, nervous and endocrine systems, which then can affect every part of your body. They really do play diverse physiological roles that influence us.

- There are many known benefits to probiotics and many more which are being discovered every day as research is fast-paced and international. These benefits affect many different bodily systems and conditions. Keeping your digestive tract as healthy as possible with probiotics and other beneficial microbes on a daily basis is the best way to prevent the consequences from an unhealthy intestinal environment.

- There are many things you are doing or taking which may be the cause of why you are probably lacking in beneficial microbes and probiotics and tipping the balance in favor of pathogenic organisms. Stop doing the unnecessary things!

- You should start slowly with probiotics and cultured foods and drinks or you may experience mild (if you are otherwise healthy) side effects as your microbiome is reconfigured. You should always check with your qualified healthcare provider if you have any concerns about probiotics.

- There are 5 major genera in the probiotics world and a few lesser others. To remember what they do, the major ones can be compared to Transformers®, security guards, police officers, Special Forces and good apples-in-the-bunch to reflect their actions. Probiotics may not dominate the GI tract in sheer numbers, but their actions can determine whether you have a healthy or unhealthy intestinal environment.

- You can find probiotics and other helpful microbes in many places. Taking them in from a variety of sources will add diversity to your GI tract. Knowing how and when to take them gives you an advantage.

- There are many important points to consider when choosing a source of probiotics, including a probiotic supplement.

By this point you must agree that the list of benefits of probiotics shown in Chapter 6 is indeed very impressive. Combine those benefits with the reasons shown in Chapter 7 of why you probably do not have enough probiotics, and you can see that it is to your advantage to consistently take probiotics and/or consume beneficial microbes in some form, and preferably several forms. Since the uniqueness of each person's communities of microbes is relatively stable over time, the only way to make changes are to consistently take the beneficial ones you don't have (or don't have enough of) and to pamper the desirable ones that you do have.

Replenishing the helpful microbes takes advantage of the fact that microbes and their genes at least equal or outnumber human cells and genes. Resistance really is futile, so you might as well work with the ones that are there to protect you and benefit you or else the opportunistic or harmful ones will dominate.

Let me backtrack a bit. As I mentioned before, I was giving my kids probiotic supplements when they were able to eat yogurt on their own. I was also taking the same supplement. In retrospect, it was probably better than taking nothing but it was too weak and too late to help me with the many autoimmune problems that had already taken hold on me without me knowing, especially since I was still eating gluten, sugars and processed foods at the time and taking multiple courses of antibiotics. I was suffering from debilitating chronic fatigue and other problems and it was not until years later that I found out I had autoimmune diseases and had absorption problems, food sensitivities and other unexplained concerns. Somehow I got started on probiotics back then and hardly ever miss a day without having either a supplement and/or some kind of beneficial-microbe food or drink. I am much, much healthier than I was then.

Some results of what happened to me I cannot change, but I try my best to use probiotics to my advantage. Note this important message: **I do not take probiotics in a vacuum, and neither should you.** Probiotics are one part of this complicated human endeavor we call *health*. You cannot eat junk, be lazy, be stressed out, not sleep well, be socially isolated and then pop a pill trying to fix it all.

What does this mean to you? Probiotics are PART of the magic bullet for health! Ensure that you get some kind of probiotic and/ or beneficial microbes daily.

Additionally, try some of these other ideas in the magic bullet:

- Start to eat more real food with real vitamins, minerals, phytonutrients, healthy fats, unaltered proteins and naturally-incorporated fiber found primarily in plant foods (and NOT found in typical Western-diet foods).
- Substantially reduce or eliminate added sugars.
- Substantially reduce or eliminate refined flours.
- Substantially reduce or eliminate artificial flavors, artificial colors, preservatives and flavor enhancers like MSG and artificial sweeteners.
- Eliminate transfats and refined vegetable oils and learn how to correctly cook with oils.
- Substantially reduce or eliminate as many over-the-counter drugs as you can.
- Talk to your healthcare provider about the medications you are taking and what, if anything, you can do to reduce your dependence on them.
- Eat organic when possible, especially for foods with soy, corn, canola, cottonseed, zucchini and yellow crookneck

squash, papaya, russet potatoes and sugar beets. Those foods are most likely GMO (genetically-modified organisms).

- Eat meat, poultry and fish that are raised the way they would naturally eat and live, not in CAFO's (confined animal feeding operations).

- Reduce stress as much as possible.

- Make sleep a priority.

- Eat more raw fruits and vegetables. *Lactobacillus plantarum* is a great probiotic species which can be found on raw produce. Fruits and vegetables have fiber and other substances which nourish you and your microbes.

- Eat more cultured/fermented foods like sauerkraut. Try some of the recipes in the next chapter.

- Drink more healthy (non-alcoholic) cultured/fermented beverages like kefir and kombucha. More information on these is provided in the next chapter.

- Drink more purified water to flush toxins out of your body, keep your cells hydrated so they can function better and keep feces moving along.

- Get your body moving so you can increase circulation, move lymph fluid and properly eliminate wastes.

By trying these ideas, you will enable foods to fulfill the positive roles they can play and your body to function the way it was intended to function. And of course, you will be using probiotics and other beneficial microbes to your advantage!

The next chapter gives you some tips and recipes to get started with fermented foods and drinks.

CHAPTER 13

Easy Recipes and Tips for Fermentation

This chapter is meant to give you a glimpse into the world of fermented (sometimes called *cultured*) foods and drinks. We have been programmed that "germs" are horrible things to be avoided, but as you have learned through this book, some microbes are not only beneficial to us buy are also essential to our survival.

Nonetheless, it can be scary starting fermentation on your own because you fear food poisoning. Fear no more! As long as you follow basic hygiene, keeping your work surface, utensils, hands and ingredients clean (wash off that carrot you dropped on the floor!), you will be fine. Never, ever eat or drink directly from the jar. Always use a clean spoon or pour the ferments into another container or you will contaminate the entire batch.

Remember that fermentation is a method of food preservation. Bacteria and yeasts transform sugars and starches in food to acids (such as lactic acid), gases or alcohol, allowing beneficial microbes to flourish and harmful ones to be killed. Fermentation can also increase the vitamins in the ferments.

Lactobacillus species of beneficial bacteria, in particular, are often present in fermented foods and drinks.

Remember, also, that it can take 10 to 16 repeated exposures before acceptance to a new food occurs.

You will see bubbles and probably smell some pungent odors as things ferment. Pungent is different than spoiled. You will know the difference between the two if you've ever smelled slimy fruits or rotting meats. However, as long as you don't see green, pink or other-colored mold, or allow your experiments to ferment so long that they are too acidic or dry out from evaporation, thus exposing the food to air, you will be fine. Remember, for most solid-food ferments, the lactic acid bacteria like *Lactobacillus* on the foods produce acids which lower the pH of the ferment. As you learned in Chapters 6 and 7, low pH kills most pathogenic microbes.

Salt also kills or inhibits the growth of pathogenic microbes, so it is used in many solid-food recipes. For solid food like vegetables, fruits, nuts and herbs, keep them under brine and you will be fine!

If ever in doubt, you can add a bit of the juice from past ferments to a new batch to quickly inoculate it.

I like to use wide-mouth quart jars for bigger batches and wide-mouth pint jars for smaller batches of solid-food ferments. The advantages of using pint jars are that you can have several different recipes fermenting at the same time, giving you a variety of foods and microbial biodiversity, and if your combination of ingredients isn't to your liking, you didn't waste much food. The downside is that you have to prepare the recipes more often. You can decide which size to use, or even if you want to use something bigger like a fermentation crock, based on your needs and preferences.

For most solid-food recipes, dry fermentation works. This involves mixing all the ingredients together and pressing them into a jar, allowing the natural juices from the ingredients to supply the liquid. For fermenting whole vegetables, fruits or nuts, you will need to supply a brine solution. This is typically one tablespoon of pink sea salt per 16 ounces of water, but may go as high as one tablespoon per 8 ounces, depending on your preference.

I recommend that you use an unrefined pink sea salt for a fuller flavor and for the trace minerals. Do not use iodized salt! It will inhibit the growth of bacteria. Remember, it is always easier to add more salt than it is to remove salt!

Many recipes call for cabbage. You may use green or purple, depending on your tastes. Purple cabbage remains crisper, but green cabbage has a sweeter, milder flavor. Some recipes have onion in them. Use mild onions and always err on the conservative side of amounts when using onions because they are very potent and can overwhelm the ferment's taste.

Try to keep your ferments at least a few feet from each other, especially if you are using cloth and a rubber band to cover the tops (such as with kombucha) in order to keep the cultures as pure as possible. If you cover your jars with solid lids, you will need to burp the jars at least once per day. To burp them, simply open them up and allow the gases to escape. You may want to keep the jars in bowls to catch any liquids which may overflow when burping.

Put something in the jar to keep the ferments submerged. Depending on the recipe, circles of large vegetables or fruits or part of a cabbage leaf or kale leaf works. You may also choose to use glass disks which I find to be very useful. If you cannot check your ferments daily, then using a cloth on the top of the jar or a specialized fermenting top which allows gases to escape may be a better option than a solid lid.

Try to use organic foods whenever possible. Although your fermenting microbes may be able to break down some of the chemicals on your foods, you want the ferments to be as beneficial as possible. Also try to use filtered water. Any chlorine residues or organic molecules in tap water are not ideal for your ferments.

Keep your culturing foods and drinks at a minimum of 55 degrees and a maximum of 75 degrees, with the exception of yogurt and kefir. Too cold and they won't culture correctly; too hot and they will ferment so quickly that you might miss the peak flavor.

Taste your cultured goods over time. While some cultured products, like yogurt or kefir, are ready in a day, relishes and veggies may be ready in as little as 3 days and as late as months in the future. Flavors and bacterial concentrations develop over time. You have to find what tastes for each recipe you prefer. When you get the result you want, refrigerate the product to slow down the fermentation. Fermentation will still proceed when the product is in the refrigerator but at a much slower pace.

How much to eat daily? As you learned in Chapter 8, it is best to start slowly when introducing microbes into your GI tract. Start with a teaspoon of cultured solids and a quarter cup or less of liquid ferments if you are new to fermentation. Remember, most cultures use fermented vegetables as condiments to meals, and even drinks like kefir and kombucha should be limited to 16 ounces per day or less. Balance, my friend, is the key to a healthy life!

By the way, don't feel like you have to be doing every ferment all the time. When I first started fermenting, I had 4 or 5 different ferments going at any given time, all in the space of my little kitchen. Keeping the jars and crocks a few feet away from each other was a challenge! Now my staple is my kombucha crock and everything else rotates in as the spirit moves me. Additionally, there is only so much room in my refrigerator and we can only eat a certain amount of food in a given time, so I've learned to temper my enthusiasm! However, at the end of the garden growing season, fermentation is an excellent way to preserve the massive amounts of produce that must be picked right before a frost and so my counters are crowded then.

Being overzealous with *anything* will surely knock your body into an imbalanced state.

There are many workshops, books, blogs and websites dedicated to fermentation. I encourage you to be adventurous and try your hand at various recipes. However, if you need a place to start or need some new ideas, these recipes and ideas are proven in my kitchen to work.

All recipes are gluten-free and dairy-free, unless you choose ingredients with those allergens.

Coconut Yogurt

I use a store-bought coconut yogurt to get my yogurt started and then use my yogurt to keep the cultures going. You could use a starter culture or even probiotic capsules if you desire. Note that since this recipe does not have additives like stabilizers or thickeners in it, the yogurt will separate into liquid and a creamier substance. Simply stir the mixture and enjoy.

- One 13.66 ounce can of full-fat coconut milk
- 1 Tablespoon of an existing coconut yogurt or use a yogurt starter culture
- 2 teaspoons coconut sugar or unrefined cane sugar

Whisk coconut milk in a small pot and slowly heat to around 180 degrees F. Whisk in coconut sugar. Let cool to around 110 degrees F. Add yogurt and whisk. Put in a glass or ceramic container and cover. Let container sit, undisturbed, in a yogurt maker, wrapped in a towel and a plant seedling mat, or in a confined space like an oven (heated for a few minutes, heat turned off and only the light on) for 8-10 hours. The target temperature for the yogurt environment is 100-115 degrees Fahrenheit. Refrigerate.

Kefir (pronounced kee'-fur or ka-feer')

You can buy kefir grains, use starter culture powder or use kefir from the store to inoculate your batch. Each has their advantages and disadvantages.

Kefir grains are like tiny cauliflower florets when activated and are a type of symbiotic culture of bacteria and yeasts (*SCOBY*). The

SCOBY will grow over time if cultivated in the proper conditions and can be gently scooped out of one finished batch of kefir and put into the next batch. The main advantage to kefir grains is that once you purchase them, they can last indefinitely if properly nourished.

The main drawback with kefir grains is that I believe you have to be a dedicated kefir maker to use the grains because they require constant exposure to new sources of nutrients. That means a daily (at most 2 days) transfer from the finished batch to the new batch. Always follow the supplier's instructions on how to prepare for the transfer.

Another drawback is that many kefir grains are meant to thrive in cow's milk, not milk alternatives like coconut, almond, soy, etc. As a result, without being occasionally refreshed in cow's milk, they will slowly lose their ability to survive.

Despite the higher maintenance of the kefir grains, using the grains and marveling at the way they transform milk into a thick, tangy drink is definitely a worthwhile experience and you may enjoy continuing it. Also, it is possible to freeze the grains if you leave town for a while. Most suppliers of the grains will provide detailed instructions on how to preserve the grains in that circumstance.

Kefir starter culture powder does not contain the same number and types of microbes as the kefir grains. No SCOBY will form when using a powder, but usually one packet of powder can be used for the first quart and then a small amount of the finished kefir can be used to inoculate the next batch, etc., for a total of 8 inoculations. Even with this method, the finished kefir should be used within a few days to inoculate the next batch and instructions for proper preparation should be followed. My website has more information on this.

Purchasing kefir is the way I think most people should start, unless you are fortunate enough to have a friend who can let you sample theirs. Since kefir is tangy, you will know if you like it or not before investing time and money into it. Be certain to buy only plain kefir, as the flavored versions usually are quite high in sugars and extra additives.

The downside is that purchased kefir is expensive compared to plain milks, but not as expensive as that coffee drink or juice bar drink you may buy! Also, purchased alternative-milk kefirs may have undesirable stabilizers in them.

For coconut milk for kefir, I use the more-liquid, unsweetened version found in a carton, and add a teaspoon of coconut sugar for each cup of kefir to give the microbes food for growth. The kefir will separate into liquid and a creamy substance, but simply shake or stir it before drinking it. My favorite way to use kefir is in a protein shake.

Hemp-Kefir Protein Shake

Hemp protein powder is a high fiber, high protein, essential fatty acid source of nutrition and is one of my favorites. Hemp protein powder is gritty, so use the amount to your liking. I prefer not to use bananas in my shakes, but bananas, nut butter or a slice of avocado can make the shake smoother.

- 3/4 cup of coconut kefir
- 3-4 Tablespoons of organic hemp protein powder
- 1 Tablespoon of good fats (coconut oil, MCT's, olive oil, hemp oil, raw nut butter)
- 1/2 cup chopped fresh or frozen greens
- 1/2 cup of fresh or frozen berries
- 1 packet of stevia
- 1/2 cup of water or less, depending on consistency

Whirl all ingredients in a blender for 20-30 seconds.

Kombucha

Kombucha is a fermented tea drink that is transformed from sweet tea to a fermented treat by a SCOBY. My website has several pages devoted to kombucha and you can definitely save a lot of money by brewing your own. I am a definite tea-lover and kombucha is one of my favorite fermented items! Here are a few recipes using plain kombucha.

Ginger Kombucha: Add 1 Tablespoon ginger juice to 8-12 ounces of kombucha.

Pomegranate Kombucha: Add 1 Tablespoon pomegranate juice to 8-12 ounces of kombucha.

Sweet Mustard Salad Dressing:

This recipe takes advantage of the microbes in kombucha and honey. Use sparingly.

- 2 Tablespoons kombucha
- 2 Tablespoons organic extra-virgin olive oil
- 1 Tablespoon Dijon mustard
- 1 Tablespoon raw unfiltered honey
- Herbs of your choice, optional

Whisk all ingredients together.

Rosemary-Kombucha Marinade

I found that I can substitute kombucha (depending on how acidic it tastes) into some marinade recipes which call for white wine. Yes, the microbes are probably killed when cooked, but the flavor is more subtle than wine and I don't have to buy white wine just for cooking anymore! This recipe is great for a marinade (enough for 18 chicken thighs) and is adapted from an old "Energy Times" recipe.

- 3/4 cup reduced sodium organic tamari
- 3/4 cup kombucha
- 1 very small onion, chopped finely
- 3 Tablespoons fresh rosemary, minced
- 3 garlic cloves, minced

Whisk ingredients together. Marinate chicken for a few hours to overnight.

Relishes and Salsas

Relishes and salsas are condiments used to add flavors to foods. Think beyond hot dogs, hamburgers and tortilla chips and use them to dress up plainly roasted meats, fish and poultry, beans and legumes, omelets, plain vegetables and plain grains such as rice or corn.

I tend to refrigerate relishes and salsas after 3 days because I like the texture and tastes at that time. However, you may certainly let them ferment longer and see when you prefer them.

Cultured Grape Salsa

This recipe is delicious served with avocado, on eggs or an omelet, with mild fish like Mahi Mahi or tilapia, with nachos or with tortilla chips as a dip.

- 5 roma tomatoes, diced (2 cups)
- About 25 red seedless grapes, cut in quarters or sixths, depending on size (1 cup)
- 1/4 purple onion, finely chopped (1/4 cup)
- 1/4 chopped cilantro
- 1/2 jalapeño pepper, minced (or more, depending on taste)
- 1 garlic clove, minced
- 2 teaspoons fresh lime juice
- 1 teaspoon unrefined pink sea salt
- 1 capsule of non-coated probiotics, opened (optional if you need a speedy fermentation)

Mix all ingredients in a glass or ceramic bowl. Transfer to a pint glass jar, gently pressing ingredients, and weigh down with something like a glass disk. Taste in 3 days and refrigerate.

Cranberry-Pomegranate Relish

This makes a great substitute for the traditional sugar-laden cooked cranberries served with turkey or mixed in a raw vegetable salad for a tangy fruit taste.

- 1/2 cup fresh or frozen cranberries
- 1/2 cup fresh or frozen pomegranate arils
- 1/2 cup chopped sweet apple
- 1/2 cup chopped orange, inner segments only
- 1 teaspoon orange zest
- 1 Tablespoon sauerkraut or other ferment juice (especially helpful when using frozen fruit)

Process all ingredients in a food processor to the desired consistency. Pack in a pint jar and weigh down with something like a glass disk. Taste in 3 days and refrigerate.

Zingy Carrot Relish

Ever notice how carrots become bitter with age? Ferment them before they reach that point and you will preserve their goodness. Scrub them but leave the skins on.

- 1 cup carrot, grated
- 1 cup parsnip, grated
- 1 cup apple, grated
- 2 teaspoons ginger, grated
- 1/2 teaspoon pink sea salt

Mix all ingredients in a glass or ceramic bowl. Transfer to a pint glass jar, packing ingredients down, and weigh down with something like a glass disk. Taste in 3 days and refrigerate.

Carrot, Ginger and Lime Relish

This adds some sweetness and zing to plain hummus.

- 1 cup carrot, grated
- 1/2 Tablespoon ginger, grated
- 1 teaspoon fresh lime juice
- 1/8 teaspoon pink sea salt

Mix all ingredients in a glass or ceramic bowl. Transfer to a pint glass jar, pressing ingredients down, and weigh down with something like a glass disk. Taste in 3 days and refrigerate.

Sauerkraut Relish

This relish is a nice addition to many meals.

- 1/4 cup red pepper, chopped
- 1/4 cup celery, chopped
- 1/4 cup onion, chopped
- 3 cups green cabbage, shredded
- ¾ teaspoon pink sea salt

Mix all ingredients in a glass or ceramic bowl. Transfer to a pint or quart glass jar, packing ingredients down, and weigh down with something like a glass disk. Taste in 3 days and refrigerate.

Longer-Cultivation Ferments

Not-Quite-Kimchi

If you are like me and are intrigued by the flavors in kimchi, but do not want raw seafood, super spiciness or the starchy paste typically used, you may like this recipe which provides flavor without the extras. There is no pre-soaking in this recipe.

- 1 head Napa cabbage. Halve, remove core and chop into 1-inch pieces
- 1 large or 2 small carrots, finely shredded (1 cup) I use unpeeled carrots
- 8 scallions, chopped (1/2 cup)
- 4 garlic cloves, minced
- 1 Tablespoon finely grated ginger
- 4 red radishes, finely shredded (1/2 cup)
- 1 Tablespoon pink sea salt
- 1 Tablespoon mild chili powder

Mix all ingredients in a glass or ceramic bowl. Transfer to quart glass jar, pressing ingredients down, and weigh down. It may fill more than one jar. Begin tasting in a few days, but allow to ferment further for flavors to develop.

String Beans and Dill

End-of-season string beans can become tough. Save the last of your summer string beans and ferment them.

Use a one quart glass jar.

- 1 green onion, minced
- 1 clove garlic, minced
- 1 Tablespoon fresh lemon juice
- 1/4 teaspoon dried dill
- 1/4 teaspoon lemon pepper
- Fresh string beans to fill jar

Add ingredients in the order listed. Cover with a brine bath of 3 cups of water with 1-1/2 Tablespoons of pink sea salt dissolved in it and cooled. Wait at least one week before tasting.

Zesty Sauerkraut

- 4 cups green cabbage, shredded
- 1/2 cup carrot, grated
- 2 radishes, grated
- 1/8 cup purple onion, chopped
- 1 garlic clove, minced
- 1/4 teaspoon celery seed
- 1 teaspoon pink sea salt (or to taste)

Mix all ingredients in a glass or ceramic bowl. Transfer to a pint or quart glass jar, packing ingredients down, and weigh down with something like a glass disk. Start tasting in 3 days but usually one week is the minimum timeframe for flavors to develop.

Mild Sauerkraut

- 4 cups green cabbage, shredded
- 1/4 teaspoon caraway seeds
- 3/4 teaspoon pink sea salt (or to taste)

Mix all ingredients in a glass or ceramic bowl. Transfer to a pint glass jar, packing ingredients down, and weigh down with something like a glass disk. Start tasting in 3 days but usually one week is the minimum timeframe for flavors to develop.

References

INTRODUCTION

1. "NIH Human Microbiome Project Defines Normal Bacterial Makeup of the Body," *National Institutes of Health*, US Dept. of Health and Human Sciences (June 13, 2012), http://www.nih.gov/news/health/jun2012/nhgri-13.htm (accessed October 29, 2012).

2. T. Olszak et al., "Microbial Exposure during Early Life Has Persistent Effects on Natural Killer T Cell Function," *Science* 336. 6080 (2012): 489-93.

3. "Human Microbiome Project," *National Institutes of Health,* US Dept. of Health and Human Sciences, http://www.commonfund.nih.gov/hmp/overview (accessed October 29, 2012).

4. "American Gut Project," *American Gut Project,* http://americangut.org/ (accessed February 2, 1014).

5. "British Gut," *British Gut,* http://www.britishgut.org/index.html (accessed February 16, 2015).

6. "Welcome," *My New Gut,* http://www.mynewgut.eu/ (accessed February 16, 2014).

7. G. Reid et al., "Harnessing Microbiome and Probiotic Research in Sub-Saharan Africa: Recommendations from an African Workshop," *Microbiome* 2.12 (2014): 1-13.

CHAPTER 1

8. "Guidelines for the Evaluation of Probiotics in Food", *World Health Organization*, Food and Agriculture Organization of the United Nations, (April 30 and May 1, 2002), http://www.who.int/foodsafety/fs_management/en/probiotic_guidelines.pdf (accessed September 15, 2011).

9. M.E. Sanders, "How Do We Know When Something Called "Probiotic" Is Really a Probiotic? A Guideline for Consumers and Health Care Professionals," *Functional Food Reviews* 1.1 (2009): 3-12.

10. D. Rachmilewitz et al., "Toll-like Receptor 9 Signaling Mediates the Anti-inflammatory Effects of Probiotics in Murine Experimental Colitis," *Gastroenterology* 126.2 (2004): 520-28.

11. "Medical Foods Guidance Documents & Regulatory Information," *FDA*, US Dept. of Health and Human Sciences, http://www.fda.gov/food/guidanceregulation/guidancedocumentsregulatoryinformation/medicalfoods/default.htm (accessed September 10, 2011).

12. C. Hill et al., "Expert Consensus Document: The International Scientific Association for Probiotics and Prebiotics Consensus Statement on the Scope and Appropriate Use of the Term Probiotic," *Nature Reviews Gastroenterology & Hepatology* 11.8 (2014): 506-14.

CHAPTER 2

13. A. Boissière et al., "Midgut Microbiota of the Malaria Mosquito Vector *Anopheles gambiae* and Interactions with *Plasmodium falciparum* Infection," *PLOS Pathogens* 8.5 (2012): 1-12.

14. "Global Probiotics in Animal Feed Market by Bacteria (Lactobacilli, Streptococcus Thermophiles, Bifidobacteria, Others), by Livestock (Cattle Feed, Poultry Feed, Swine Feed, Pet Food), by Geography – Analysis & Forecast to 2019," *MicroMarketMonitor*, (July, 2015), http://www.micromarketmonitor.com/market-report/probiotics-in-animal-feed-reports-5329602333.html (accessed July, 16, 2015).

15. "Top 10 Vet Visit Reasons for Dogs and Cats," *Veterinary Practice News,* http://www.veterinarypracticenews.com/May-2014/Top-10-Vet-Visit-Reasons-For-Dogs-And-Cats/ (accessed September 3, 2015).

16. S. Wang et al., "Fighting malaria with engineered symbiotic bacteria from vector mosquitoes," *PNAS* 109.31 (2012): 12734-739.

17. "Of mice and men – Are mice relevant models for human disease?" *European Commission,* (May 21, 2010), http://ec.europa.eu/research/health/pdf/summary-report-25082010_en.pdf (accessed May 18, 2015).

CHAPTER 3

18. I. Moreno-Indias et al., "Impact of the Gut Microbiota on the Development of Obesity and Type 2 Diabetes Mellitus," *Frontiers in Microbiology* 5.190 (2014): 1-10.

19. "Instructions to Authors," *Journal of Bacteriology,* http://jb.asm.org/site/misc/journal-ita_nom.xhtml (accessed November 3, 2012).

CHAPTER 4

20. "NIH Human Microbiome Project Defines Normal Bacterial Makeup of the Body," *National Institutes of Health* (June, 2012), http://www.nih.gov/news/health/jun2012/nhgri-13.htm (accessed April 4, 2014).

21. J. Qin et al., "A Human Gut Microbial Gene Catalogue Established by Metagenomic Sequencing," *Nature,* 464 (2010): 59-65.

22. R. Sender et al., "Revised Estimates for the Number of Human and Bacteria Cells in the Body," BioRxiv, http://biorxiv.org/content/early/2016/01/06/036103 (accessed January 7, 2016).

23. M.B. Miller et al., "Quorum Sensing in Bacteria," *Annual Reviews Microbiology* 55 (2001): 165-99.

24. M. Baruch et al., "An Extracellular Bacterial Pathogen Modulates Host Metabolism to Regulate Its Own Sensing and Proliferation," *Cell* 156.1-2 (2014): 97-108.

25. B. Lasarre et al., "Exploiting Quorum Sensing To Confuse Bacterial Pathogens," *Microbiology and Molecular Biology Reviews* 77.1 (2013): 73-111.

26. "Research on Microbial Biofilms," *National Institutes of Health,* Grants, (December, 2002), http://grants.nih.gov/grants/guide/pa-files/PA-03-047. html (accessed September 25, 2011).

27. "Bacterial 'Bunches' Linked to Some Colorectal Cancers," *John Hopkins Medicine,* http://www.hopkinsmedicine.org/news/media/releases/bacterial_ bunches_linked_to_some_colorectal_cancers (accessed December 31, 2014).

28. H.F. Helander et al., "Surface Area of the Digestive Tract – Revisited," *Scandinavian Journal of Gastroenterology* 49.6 (2014): 681-89.

29. W.L. Hao et al., "Microflora of the Gastrointestinal Tract: A Review," *Methods in Molecular Biology* 268 (2004): 491-502.

30. S.J. Ott et al., "Quantification of Intestinal Bacterial Populations by Real-Time PCR with a Universal Primer Set and Minor Groove Binder Probes: A Global Approach to the Enteric Flora," *Journal of Clinical Microbiology* 42.6 (2004): 2566-572.

31. R.A. Bowen et al., "Microbial Life in the Digestive Tract," *Pathophysiology of the Digestive System.* Colorado State University (July, 2006), http://www. vivo.colostate.edu/hbooks/pathphys/digestion/index.html (accessed February 28, 2012).

32. W. Landers, "Oral Bacteria: How Many? How Fast?" *RDH.* PennWell Corporation, http://www.rdhmag.com/articles/print/volume-29/issue-7/ columns/the-landers-file/oral-bacteria-how-many-how-fast.html (accessed September 14, 2014).

33. J.C. Stearns et al., "Bacterial Biogeography of the Human Digestive Tract," *Scientific Reports* 170.1 (2011): 1-9.

34. X.C. Morgan et al., "Dysfunction of the Intestinal Microbiome in Inflammatory Bowel Disease and Treatment," *Genome Biology* 13.9 (2012): 1-18.

35. A. Durbán et al., "Assessing Gut Microbial Diversity from Feces and Rectal Mucosa," *Microbial Ecology* 61.1 (2010): 123-33.

36. M. Sharbatdaran et al., "Comparison of Stool Antigen with Gastric Biopsy for the Detection of *Helicobacter pylori* Infection," *Pakistan Journal of Medical Sciences* 29.1 (2013): 68-71.

37. E. Papa et al., "Non-Invasive Mapping of the Gastrointestinal Microbiota Identifies Children with Inflammatory Bowel Disease," *PLoS ONE* 7.6 (2012): E39242.

38. Y. Momozawa et al., "Characterization of Bacteria in Biopsies of Colon and Stools by High Throughput Sequencing of the V2 Region of Bacterial 16S RRNA Gene in Human," *PLoS ONE* 6.2 (2011): E16952.

39. "Feces," *Encyclopedia Britannica Online,* http://www.britannica.com/EBchecked/topic/203293/feces (accessed October 28, 2014).

CHAPTER 5

40. G. Vigni et al., "Allergy and the Gastrointestinal System." *Clinical & Experimental Immunology* 153 (2008): 3-6.

41. Parham, Peter. *The Immune System*. New York: Garland Science, 2009. Print.

42. Y. Goto et al., "Epithelial Barrier: An Interface for the Cross-communication between Gut Flora and Immune System," *Immunological Reviews* 245.1 (2012): 147-63.

43. H. Konishi et al., "Traffic Control of Bacteria-Derived Molecules: A New System of Host-Bacterial Crosstalk," *International Journal of Cell Biology* 2013 (2013): 1-8.

44. M-H Wang et al., "A Novel Approach to Detect Cumulative Genetic Effects and Genetic Interactions in Crohn's Disease," *Inflammatory Bowel Diseases* 19.9 (2013): 1799-1808.

45. "Ulcerative colitis," *University of Maryland Medical Center* (December 21, 2012), http://umm.edu/health/medical/reports/articles/ulcerative-colitis (accessed on October 21, 2014).

46. K. Fischer, "Gene Marker Predicts Celiac Disease Risk in Young Children," *Healthline*. Healthline Networks (July 2, 2014), http://www.

healthline.com/health-news/gene-predicts-celiac-risk-070214 (accessed on October 21, 2014).

47. "Celiac Disease: Who Is at Risk?" *National Foundation for Celiac Disease Awareness,* http://www.celiaccentral.org/riskfactors/ (accessed on October 21, 2014).

48. G.D. Wu, "Non-bacterial Microbes in the Gut: What Are They, How Do We Characterize Them, and What Do They Do?" GMFH 2014 Summit. Florida, Miami. (March 28, 2014). Lecture.

49. K.E. Fujimura et al., "Role of the Gut Microbiota in Defining Human Health," *Expert Review of Anti-infective Therapy* 8.4 (2010): 435-54.

50. R. Lewis, "Microbiome Adapts to Diet Change in a Day," *Medscape Medical News,* WebMD (December 12, 2013), http://www.medscape.com/viewarticle/817769 (accessed on December 14, 2013).

51. C. Bergland, "How Does the Vagus Nerve Convey Gut Instincts to the Brain?" Web log post. *Psychology Today* (May 23, 2014), http://www.psychologytoday.com/blog/the-athletes-way/201405/how-does-the-vagus-nerve-convey-gut-instincts-the-brain (accessed July 21, 2014).

52. A. Hadhazy. "Think Twice: How the Gut's "Second Brain" Influences Mood and Well-Being," *Scientific American* (February 10, 2012), http://www.scientificamerican.com/article/gut-second-brain/ (accessed April 20, 2014).

53. F-C Hsieh et al., "Oral Administration of *Lactobacillus reuteri* GMNL-263 Improves Insulin Resistance and Ameliorates Hepatic Steatosis in High Fructose-fed Rats," *Nutrition & Metabolism* 10.35 (2013): 1-14.

CHAPTER 6

54. F. Kunst et al., "The complete genome sequence of the Gram-positive bacterium *Bacillus subtilis*," *Nature* 390 (1997): 249-56.

55. "Gram-negative Bacteria Infections in Healthcare Settings," *Centers for Disease Control and Prevention* (January 17, 2011), http://www.cdc.gov/hai/organisms/gram-negative-bacteria.html (accessed June 28, 2014).

56. *Medical Microbiology, 4th edition.* Baron S, editor. Galveston (TX): University of Texas Medical Branch at Galveston; 1996. Print.

57. G.D. Wu, "Non-bacterial Microbes in the Gut: What Are They, How Do We Characterize Them, and What Do They Do?" GMFH 2014 Summit. Florida, Miami. (March 28, 2014). Lecture.

58. H. Xu et al., "Assessment of Cell Surface Properties and Adhesion Potential of Selected Probiotic Strains," *Letters in Applied Microbiology* 49.4 (2009): 434-42.

59. S. Fujiwara et al., "Purification and Characterization of a Novel Protein Produced by *Bifidobacterium longum* SBT2928 That Inhibits the Binding of Enterotoxigenic *Escherichia coli* Pb176 (CFA/II) to Galgliotetraosylceramide," *Journal of Applied Microbiology* 86.4 (1999): 615-21.

60. J. Woo et al., "Probiotic-mediated Competition, Exclusion and Displacement in Biofilm Formation by Food-borne Pathogens," *Letters in Applied Microbiology* 56.4 (2013): 307-13.

61. K.Y. Wang et al., "Effects of Ingesting *Lactobacillus*- and *Bifidobacterium*-containing Yogurt in Subjects with Colonized *Helicobacter pylori*," *The American Journal of Clinical Nutrition* 80.3 (2004): 737-41.

62. V. Cleusix et al., "Inhibitory Activity Spectrum of Reuterin Produced by *Lactobacillus reuteri* against Intestinal Bacteria," *BMC Microbiology* 7.101 (2007): 1-9.

63. B. Deplancke et al., "Microbial Modulation of Innate Defense: Goblet Cells and the Intestinal Mucus Layer," *American Journal of Clinical Nutrition* 73.6 (2001): 11315-1415.

64. J.M. Laparra et al., "*Bifidobacterium longum* CECT 7347 Modulates Immune Responses in a Gliadin-Induced Enteropathy Animal Model," *PLoS ONE* 7.2 (2012): E30744.

65. S.E. Gilliland et al., "Deconjugation of Bile Acids by Intestinal Lactobacilli," *Applied and Environmental Microbiology* 33.1 (1977): 15-18.

66. F. Yan et al., "Probiotics: Progress toward Novel Therapies for Intestinal Diseases," *Current Opinion in Gastroenterology* 26.2 (2010): 95-101.

67. I.C. Arts et al., "Polyphenols and Disease Risk in Epidemiologic Studies," *The American Journal of Clinical Nutrition* 81.1 (2005): 317S-25S.

68. K.E. Fujimura et al., "Role of the Gut Microbiota in Defining Human Health," *Expert Review of Anti-infective Therapy* 8.4 (2010): 435-54.

69. M.Z. Cader et al., "Recent Advances in Inflammatory Bowel Disease: Mucosal Immune Cells in Intestinal Inflammation," *BMJ* 62 (2013): 1653-664.

70. N.C. Reading et al., "The Starting Lineup: Key Microbial Players in Intestinal Immunity and Homeostasis," *Frontiers in Cellular and Infection Microbiology* 2.148 (2011): 1-10.

71. J.Z. Xiao et al., "Effect of Probiotic *Bifidobacterium longum* BBS36 in Relieving Clinical Symptoms and Modulating Plasma Cytokine Levels of Japanese Cedar Pollinosis during the Pollen Season. A Randomized Double-blind, Placebo-controlled Trial," *Journal of Investigational Allergology and Clinical Immunology* 16.2 (2006): 86-93.

72. E. Larsson et al., "Analysis of Gut Microbial Regulation of Host Gene Expression along the Length of the Gut and Regulation of Gut Microbial Ecology through MyD88," *Gut* 61 (2012): 1124-131.

73. G. Reuter, "The *Lactobacillus* and *Bifidobacterium* Microflora of the Human Intestine: Composition and Succession," *Current Issues in Intestinal Microbiology* 2.2 (2001): 43-53.

74. F. Yan et al., "Probiotics: Progress toward Novel Therapies for Intestinal Diseases," *Current Opinion in Gastroenterology* 26.2 (2010): 95-101.

75. D. Groeger et al., "*Bifidobacterium infantis* 35624 Modulates Host Inflammatory Processes beyond the Gut," *Gut Microbes* 4.4 (2013): 325-39.

76. M. Ventura et al., "Genome-Scale Analyses of Health-Promoting Bacteria: Probiogenomics," *Nature Reviews Microbiology* 7.1 (2008): 61-71.

77. S.H. Al-Sheraji et al., "Hypocholesterolaemic Effect of Yoghurt Containing *Bifidobacterium pseudocatenulatum* G4 or *Bifidobacterium longum* BB536," *Food Chemistry* 135.2 (2012): 356-61.

78. M. Stojančević et al., "The Influence of Intestinal Tract and Probiotics on the Fate of Orally Administered Drugs," *Current Issues in Molecular Biology* 16 (2014): 55-68.

79. M. Rossi et al., "Folate Production by Probiotic Bacteria," *Nutrients* 3.1 (2011): 118-34.

80. P. Marteau et al., "*Bifidobacterium animalis* strain DN-173 010 shortens the colonic transit time in healthy women: a double-blind, randomized, controlled study," *Alimentary Pharmacology and Therapeutics* 16.3 (2002): 587-93.

81. H.J. Krammer et al., "Effect of *Lactobacillus casei* Shirota on Colonic Transit Time in Patients with Chronic Constipation," *Coloproctology* 33.2 (2011): 109-13.

82. P. Marteau et al., "*Bifidobacterium animalis* strain DN-173 010 shortens the colonic transit time in healthy women: a double-blind, randomized, controlled study," *Alimentary Pharmacology and Therapeutics* 16.3 (2002): 587-93.

83. A. Chmielewska et al., "Systematic Review of Randomised Controlled Trials: Probiotics for Functional Constipation," *World Journal of Gastroenterology* 16.1 (2010): 69-75.

84. R. Pattani et al., "Probiotics for the Prevention of Antibiotic-Associated Diarrhea and *Clostridium difficile* Infection among Hospitalized Patients: Systematic Review and Meta-analysis," *Open Medicine.* 7.2 (2013): e56-e67.

85. G. Grandy et al., "Probiotics in the Treatment of Acute Rotavirus Diarrhoea. A Randomized, Double-blind, Controlled Trial Using Two Different Probiotic Preparations in Bolivian Children," *BMC Infectious Diseases* 10.253 (2010): 1-7.

86. C. Dunne et al., "In Vitro Selection Criteria for Probiotic Bacteria of Human Origin: Correlation with in Vivo Findings," *Gut* 61 (2012): 1124-131.

87. L.R. Fitzpatrick, "Probiotics for the Treatment of *Clostridium difficile* Associated Disease," *World Journal of Gastrointestinal Pathophysiology* 4.3 (2013): 47-52.

88. F. Indrio et al., "Prophylactic Use of a Probiotic in the Prevention of Colic, Regurgitation, and Functional Constipation," *JAMA Pediatrics* 168.3 (2014): 228-33.

89. T.M. Frech et al., "Probiotics for the Treatment of Systemic Sclerosis-associated Gastrointestinal Bloating/ Distention," *Clinical and Experimental Rheumatology Online* 29.2 (2011): S22-S25.

90. T. Mimura et al., "Once Daily High Dose Probiotic Therapy (VSL#3) for Maintaining Remission in Recurrent or Refractory Pouchitis," *Gut* 53 (2004): 108-114.

91. J.M. Bixquert, "Treatment of Irritable Bowel Syndrome with Probiotics: An Etiopathogenic Approach at Last?" *Revista Española De Enfermedades Digestivas* 101.8 (2009): 553-64.

92. L. Hun, "Original Research: *Bacillus coagulans* Significantly Improved Abdominal Pain and Bloating in Patients with IBS," *Postgraduate Medicine* 121.2 (2009): 119-24.

CHAPTER 7

93. "The Earliest Alcoholic Beverage in the World," *Penn Museum*. University of Pennsylvania Museum of Archaeology and Anthropology, http://www.penn.museum/research/research-asian-section/783-the-earliest-alcoholic-beverage-in-the-world.html (accessed November 5, 2013).

94. N.F. Haard NF et al., *Fermented Cereals: A Global Perspective*. Rome: Food and Agriculture Organization of the United Nations, 1999. Print.

95. "Slow Food," *Slow Food*, http://www.slowfood.com (accessed April 20, 2009).

96. "The Weston A. Price Foundation – Home," *The Weston A. Price Foundation for Wise Traditions in Food, Farming and the Healing Arts,* http://www.westonaprice.org/ (accessed April 20, 2009).

97. L.A. Knodler, "Dissemination of Invasive *Salmonella* via Bacterial-induced Extrusion of Mucosal Epithelia," *PNAS* 107.41 (2010): 17733-7738.

98. D.B. Lowrie et al., "Division and Death Rates of *Salmonella typhimurium* Inside Macrophages: Use of Penicillin as a Probe, *Microbiology* 110.2 (1979): 409-19.

99. M.P. Zacharof et al., "Optimization of Growth Conditions for Intensive Propagation, Growth Development and Lactic Acid Production of Selected Strains of Lactobacilli," *Engineering Our Future: Are We up to the Challenge?* Proc. of Chemeca 2009, Australia, Perth. 2009. 1830-838, http://search.informit.com.au/documentSummary;dn=797622581798127;res=IELENG (accessed July 6, 2014).

100. Y.K. Lee et al., "Permanent Colonization by *Lactobacillus casei* is Hindered by the Low Rate of Cell Division in Mouse Gut," *Applied and Environmental Microbiology* 70.2 (2004): 670-74.

101. J. Suez et al., "Artificial Sweeteners Induce Glucose Intolerance by Altering the Gut Microbiota," *Nature* (2014): 181-86.

102. S.S. Schiffman et al., "Sucralose, A Synthetic Organochlorine Sweetener: Overview of Biological Issues," *Journal of Toxicology and Environmental Health, Part B* 16.7 (2013): 399-451.

103. M.B. Abou-Donia et al., "Splenda Alters Gut Microflora and Increases Intestinal P-Glycoprotein and Cytochrome P-450 in Male Rats," *Journal of Toxicology and Environmental Health, Part A* 71.21 (2008): 1415-429.

104. D. Brusick et al., "Expert Panel Report on a Study of Splenda in Male Rats," *Regulatory Toxicology and Pharmacology* 55.1 (2009): 6-12.

105. A. Mallett et al., "Modification of Rat Caecal Microbial Biotransformation Activities by Dietary Saccharin," *Toxicology* 36.2-3 (1985): 253-62.

106. G.D. Wu et al., "Linking Long-Term Dietary Patterns with Gut Microbial Enterotypes," *Science* 334.6052 (2011): 105-08.

107. "2014 National Diabetes Statistics Report," *Centers for Disease Control and Prevention* (May 15, 2015), http://www.cdc.gov/diabetes/data/statistics/2014statisticsreport.html (accessed June 8, 2015).

108. "Therapeutic Drug Use," *Centers for Disease Control and Prevention.* (May 15, 2015), http://www.cdc.gov/nchs/fastats/drug-use-therapeutic.htm (accessed on November 13, 2015)

109. H. Cederlund et al., "Antibacterial Activities of Non-antibiotic Drugs," *Journal of Antimicrobial Chemotherapy* 32.3 (1993): 355-65.

110. J.E. Anderson, "Nutrition and Oral Contraceptives," Colorado State University Extension (December, 2010), http://www.ext.colostate.edu/pubs/foodnut/09323.html (accessed November 4, 2014).

111. R.D. Pridmore et al., "The Genome Sequence of the Probiotic Intestinal Bacterium *Lactobacillus johnsonii* NCC 533," PNAS 101.8 (2004): 2512-517.

112. F. Fouhy et al., "High-Throughput Sequencing Reveals the Incomplete, Short-Term Recovery of Infant Gut Microbiota following Parenteral Antibiotic Treatment with Ampicillin and Gentamicin," *Antimicrobial Agents and Chemotherapy* 56.11 (2012): 5811-820.

113. "FDA Approves Two Therapies to Treat IBS-D," *U.S. Food and Drug Administration*, US Dept. of Health and Human Services (May 27, 2015), http://www.fda.gov/NewsEvents/Newsroom/PressAnnouncements/ucm448328.htm (accessed June 3, 2015).

114. "FDA's Strategy on Antimicrobial Resistance - Questions and Answers," *FDA*. U.S. Department of Health and Human Services (June 11, 2015), http://www.fda.gov/AnimalVeterinary/GuidanceComplianceEnforcement/GuidanceforIndustry/ucm216939.htm (accessed November 13, 2015).

115. M.A.M. Rogers et al., "Depression, Antidepressant Medications, and Risk of *Clostridium difficile* Infection," *BMC Medicine* 11.1 (2013): 121.

116. C. Lass-Flörl, "Antifungal Properties of Selective Serotonin Reuptake Inhibitors against *Aspergillus* Species *In Vitro*," *Journal of Antimicrobial Chemotherapy* 48.6 (2001): 775-79.

117. R. Kaufman, "Prozac Killing *E. coli* in the Great Lakes," *National Geographic*. National Geographic Society (May 25, 2011), http://news.nationalgeographic.com/news/2011/05/11052-prozac-drugs-water-great-lakes-erie/ (accessed November 7, 2014).

118. US Dept. of Health and Human Sciences, FDA, *Fish and Fishery Products Hazards and Controls Guidance - Fourth Edition*, http://www.fda.gov/food/guidanceregulation/guidancedocumentsregulatoryinformation/seafood/ucm2018426.htm (accessed February 3, 2013).

119. A. Lanas et al., "Nonsteroidal Anti-Inflammatory Drugs and Lower Gastrointestinal Complications," *Gastroenterology Clinics of North America* 38.2 (2009): 333-52.

120. L. Montenegro et al., "Non-Steroidal Anti-inflammatory Drug Induced Damage on Lower Gastro-intestinal Tract: Is There an Involvement of Microbiota?" *Current Drug Safety* 9.3 (2014): 196-204.

121. S. Syer et al., "NSAID Enteropathy and Bacteria: A Complicated Relationship," *Journal of Gastroenterology* 50.4 (2015): 387-93.

122. U. Titilayo et al., "Antimicrobial Activity of Non-steroidal Anti-inflammatory Drugs with Respect to Immunological Response: Diclofenac Sodium as a Case Study," *African Journal of Biotechnology* 8.25 (2009): 7332-339.

123. E. Schonbrunn et al., "Interaction of the Herbicide Glyphosate with Its Target Enzyme 5-enolpyruvylshikimate 3-phosphate Synthase in Atomic Detail," *Proceedings of the National Academy of Sciences* 98.4 (2001): 1376-380.

124. W. Lu et al., "Genome-wide Transcriptional Responses of *Escherichia coli* to Glyphosate, a Potent Inhibitor of the Shikimate Pathway Enzyme 5-enolpyruvylshikimate-3-phosphate Synthase," *Molecular BioSystems* 9.3 (2013): 522-30.

125. A.A. Shehata et al., "The Effect of Glyphosate on Potential Pathogens and Beneficial Members of Poultry Microbiota *In Vitro*," *Current Microbiology* 66.4 (2012): 350-58.

126. M. Krüger et al., "Detection of Glyphosate Residues in Animals and Humans," *Journal of Environmental & Analytical Toxicology* 4.2 (2014): 1-5.

127. T. Bøhn et al., "Compositional Differences in Soybeans on the Market: Glyphosate Accumulates in Roundup Ready GM Soybeans," *Food Chemistry* 153 (2014): 207-15.

128. B. Kurenbach et al., "Sublethal Exposure to Commercial Formulations of the Herbicides Dicamba, 2,4-Dichlorophenoxyacetic Acid, and Glyphosate Cause Changes in Antibiotic Susceptibility in *Escherichia coli* and *Salmonella enterica* Serovar Typhimurium," *MBio* 6.2 (2015): 1-9.

129. R. Mesnage et al., "Cytotoxicity on Human Cells of Cry1Ab and Cry1Ac Bt Insecticidal Toxins Alone or with a Glyphosate-based Herbicide," *Journal of Applied Toxicology* 33.7 (2012): 695-99.

130. "IARC Monographs on the Evaluation of Carcinogenic Risks to Humans," *IARC Monographs* (March 20, 2015), http://monographs.iarc.fr/ENG/Monographs/vol112/index.php (accessed March 22, 2015).

131. G. Reid et al., "Harnessing Microbiome and Probiotic Research in Sub-Saharan Africa: Recommendations from an African Workshop," *Microbiome* 2.12 (2014): 1-13.

132. C.A. Thaiss et al., "Transkingdom Control of Microbiota Diurnal Oscillations Promotes Metabolic Homeostasis," *Cell* 159.3 (2014): 514-29.

133. J. Henao-Mejia et al., "Microbiota Keep the Intestinal Clock Ticking," *Cell* 153.4 (2013): 741-43.

134. "Fact Sheet on Stress." *NIMH*. National Institute of Mental Health, http://www.nimh.nih.gov/health/publications/stress/index.shtml (accessed December 7, 2014).

135. S.X. Wang et al., "Effects of Psychological Stress on Small Intestinal Motility and Bacteria and Mucosa in Mice," *World Journal of Gastroenterology* 11.13 (2005): 2016-021.

136. S.R. Knowles et al., "Investigating the Role of Perceived Stress on Bacterial Flora Activity and Salivary Cortisol Secretion: A Possible Mechanism Underlying Susceptibility to Illness," *Biological Psychology* 77.2 (2008): 132-37.

CHAPTER 8

137. "The Jarisch-Herxheimer Reaction," *The Lancet* 309.8007 (1977): 340-41.

138. M.E. Sanders, "How Do We Know When Something Called "Probiotic" Is Really a Probiotic? A Guideline for Consumers and Health Care Professionals," *Functional Food Reviews* 1.1 (2009): 3-12.

CHAPTER 9

139. H.A. Hong et al., "Defining the Natural Habitat of *Bacillus* Spore-formers," *Research in Microbiology* 160.6 (2009): 375-79.

140. N.K. Tam et al., "The Intestinal Life Cycle of *Bacillus subtilis* and Close Relatives," *Journal of Bacteriology* 188.7 (2006): 2692-700.

141. I. Sorokulova, "Modern Status and Perspectives of *Bacillus* Bacteria as Probiotics," *Journal of Probiotics & Health* 1.4 (2013): 1-5.

142. P. Permpoonpattana et al., "Evaluation of *Bacillus subtilis* Strains as Probiotics and Their Potential as a Food Ingredient," *Beneficial Microbes* 3.2 (2012): 127-35.

143. Sarles, W.B. and B.W. Hammer, "Observations on *Bacillus coagulans,*" *Journal of Bacteriology.* 23.4 (1932): 301-14.

144. D.H. Bergey et al., *Manual of Determinative Bacteriology.* Baltimore, Md: Williams & Wilkins, 1957. Print.

145. M.E. Sanders et al., "Sporeformers as Human Probiotics: *Bacillus, Sporolactobacillus,* and *Brevibacillus,*" *Comprehensive Reviews in Food Science and Food Safety,* 2 (2003): 101-10.

146. H. Schulz, "Sabinsa Widening Horizons for Probiotic Ingredient," *NutraIngredients-USA.com,* (October 4, 2012), http://www.nutraingredients-usa.com/Suppliers2/Sabinsa-widening-horizons-for-probiotic-ingredient (accessed December 6, 2013).

147. D.M. Keefe, "Agency Response Letter GRAS Notice No. GRN 000399", *USA. FDA.* Office of Food Additive Safety (July 31, 2012), http://www.fda.gov/Food/IngredientsPackagingLabeling/GRAS/NoticeInventory/ucm314145.htm (accessed November 6, 2013).

148. D.F Ohye, "Formation and Structure of the Spore of *Bacillus coagulans,*" *The Journal of Cell Biology* 14.1 (1962): 111-23.

149. USA. FDA. *Notice to US Food and Drug Administration That Bacillus coagulans GBI-30, 6086, a Novel Probiotic, Is Generally Recognized as Safe for Use in Foods.* Mayfield Heights: Ganeden Biotech, 2011. Print.

150. M.S. Rhee, et al., "Complete Genome Sequence of a Thermotolerant Sporogenic Lactic Acid Bacterium, *Bacillus coagulans* strain 36D1," *Standards in Genomic Sciences*, 5.3 (2011): 331-40.

151. F. Kunst et al., "The Complete Genome Sequence of the Gram-Positive Bacterium *Bacillus subtilis*," *Nature* 390 (1997): 249-56.

152. A. Matarante et al., "Genotyping and Toxigenic Potential of *Bacillus subtilis* and *Bacillus pumilus* Strains Occurring in Industrial and Artisanal Cured Sausages," *Applied and Environmental Microbiology* 70.9 (2004): 5168-176.

153. C. From et al., "Toxin-Producing Ability among *Bacillus* spp. Outside the *Bacillus cereus* Group," *Applied and Environmental Microbiology*, 71.3 (2005): 1178-183.

154. "*Bacillus subtilis* Final Risk Assessment," *EPA*. Environmental Protection Agency (September 27, 2012), http://www.epa.gov/biotech_rule/pubs/fra/fra009.htm (accessed November 6, 2013).

155. L.H. Duc et al., "Characterization of *Bacillus* Probiotics Available for Human Use," *Applied and Environmental Microbiology* 70.4 (2004): 2161-171.

156. V. Barbe et al., "From a Consortium Sequence to a Unified Sequence: The *Bacillus subtilis* 168 Reference Genome a Decade Later," *Microbiology* 155.6 (2009): 1758-775.

157. I.V. Pinchuk et al., "*In Vitro* Anti-*Helicobacter pylori* Activity of the Probiotic Strain *Bacillus subtilis* 3 Is Due to Secretion of Antibiotics," *Antimicrobial Agents and Chemotherapy*, 45.11 (2001): 3156-161.

158. B.R. Belitsky, "Physical and Enzymological Interaction of *Bacillus subtilis* Proteins Required for De Novo Pyridoxal 5'-Phosphate Biosynthesis," *Journal of Bacteriology* 186.4 (2004): 1191-196.

159. J-M Huang et al., "Immunostimulatory Activity of Bacillus Spores," *FEMS Immunology & Medical Microbiology* 53 (2008): 195-203.

160. R. Bentley et al., "Biosynthesis of vitamin K (menaquinone) in bacteria," *Microbiological Reviews*, 46.3 (1982): 241-80.

161. A.S Naidu et al., "Probiotic Spectra of Lactic Acid Bacteria (LAB)," *Critical Reviews in Food Science and Nutrition* 39.1 (1999): 13-126.

162. G. Reuter, "The *Lactobacillus* and *Bifidobacterium* Microflora of the Human Intestine: Composition and Succession," *Current Issues in Intestinal Microbiology* 2.2 (2001): 43-53.

163. M. Ventura et al., "Genome-Scale Analyses of Health-Promoting Bacteria: Probiogenomics." *Nature Reviews Microbiology* 7.1 (2008): 61-71.

164. N.C. Reading et al., "The Starting Lineup: Key Microbial Players in Intestinal Immunity and Homeostasis," *Frontiers in Cellular and Infection Microbiology* 2.148 (2011): 1-10.

165. F. Yan et al., "Probiotics: Progress toward Novel Therapies for Intestinal Diseases," *Current Opinion in Gastroenterology* 26.2 (2010): 95-101.

166. R. Van Der Meulen et al., "Kinetic Analysis of Bifidobacterial Metabolism Reveals a Minor Role of Succinic Acid in the Regeneration of NAD+ through Its Growth-Associated Production," *Applied and Environmental Microbiology* 72.8 (2006): 5204-210.

167. V. Lievin et al, "*Bifidobacterium* Strains from Resident Infant Human Gastrointestinal Microflora Exert Antimicrobial Activity," *Gut* 47.5 (2000): 646-52.

168. C. Dunne et al., "In Vitro Selection Criteria for Probiotic Bacteria of Human Origin: Correlation with in Vivo Findings," *Gut* 61 (2012): 1124-131.

169. M.A. Schell et al., "The Genome Sequence of *Bifidobacterium longum* Reflects Its Adaptation to the Human Gastrointestinal Tract," *PNAS* 99.22 (2002): 14422-427.

170. M. Rossi et al., "Folate Production by Probiotic Bacteria," *Nutrients* 3.1 (2011): 118-34.

171. S. Guglielmetti et al., "Randomised Clinical Trial: *Bifidobacterium bifidum* MIMBb75 Significantly Alleviates Irritable Bowel Syndrome and Improves Quality of Life--a Double-blind, Placebo-controlled Study," *Alimentary Pharmacology & Therapeutics* 33.10 (2011): 1123-132.

172. K.E. Fujimura et al., "Role of the Gut Microbiota in Defining Human Health," *Expert Review of Anti-infective Therapy* 8.4 (2010): 435-54.

173. B. Mayo and D Van Sinderen, eds. *Bifidobacteria: Genomics and Molecular Aspects.* Norfolk, UK: Caister Academic, 2010. Print.

174. R. Campana et al., "Antagonistic Activity of *Lactobacillus acidophilus* ATCC 4356 on the Growth and Adhesion/invasion Characteristics of Human *Campylobacter jejuni*," *Current Microbiology* 64.4 (2012): 371-78.

175. P.K. Gopal et al., "In Vitro Adherence Properties of *Lactobacillus rhamnosus* DR20 and *Bifidobacterium lactis* DR10 Strains and Their Antagonistic Activity against an Enterotoxigenic *Escherichia coli*," *International Journal of Food Microbiology* 67.3 (2001): 207-16.

176. S. Resta-Lenert et al., "Live Probiotics Protect Intestinal Epithelial Cells from the Effects of Infection with Enteroinvasive *Escherichia coli* (EIEC)," *Gut* 52.7 (2003): 988-97.

177. Fisher, K. "Lactose Hydrolyzing Enzymes in *Lactobacillus acidophilus* Strains," *Food Microbiology* 2.1 (1985): 23-29.

178. U. Farooq et al., "Enhancement of Short Chain Fatty Acid Production from Millet Fibres by Pure Cultures of Probiotic Fermentation," *Tropical Journal of Pharmaceutical Research* 12.2 (2013): 189-94.

179. M.S. Turner et al., "Inhibition of *Staphylococcus aureus* Growth on Tellurite-Containing Media by *Lactobacillus reuteri* Is Dependent on CyuC and Thiol Production," *Applied Environmental Microbiology*, 73.3 (2007): 1005-1009.

180. D.A. Eschenbach et al., "Prevalence of Hydrogen Peroxide-producing *Lactobacillus* Species in Normal Women and Women with Bacterial Vaginosis," *Journal of Clinical Microbiology* 27.2 (1989): 251-56.

181. I.A. Casas et al., "Validation of the Probiotic Concept: *Lactobacillus reuteri* Confers Broad-spectrum Protection against Disease in Humans and Animals," *Microbial Ecology in Health & Disease* 12.4 (2000): 247-85.

182. Y. Chiba et al., "Well-controlled Proinflammatory Cytokine Responses of Peyer's Patch Cells to Probiotic *Lactobacillus casei*," *Immunology* 130.3 (2010): 352-62.

183. E.M. Fernandez et al., "Anti-inflammatory Capacity of Selected Lactobacilli in Experimental Colitis Is Driven by NOD2-mediated

Recognition of a Specific Peptidoglycan-derived Muropeptide," *Gut* 60.8 (2011): 1050-059.

184. D.M. Saulnier et al., "The Intestinal Microbiome, Probiotics and Prebiotics in Neurogastroenterology," *Gut Microbes* 4.1 (2013): 17-27.

185. E.C. Dinleyici et al., "Clinical Efficacy of *Saccharomyces boulardii* and Metronidazole Compared to Metronidazole Alone in Children with Acute Bloody Diarrhea Caused by Amebiasis: A Prospective, Randomized, Open Label Study," *American Journal of Tropical Medicine and Hygiene* 80.6 (2009): 953-55.

186. B.A. Besirbellioglu et al., "*Saccharomyces boulardii* and Infection Due to *Giardia Lamblia,*" *Scandinavian Journal of Infectious Diseases* 38.6-7 (2006): 479-81.

187. R. Berg et al., "Inhibition of *Candida albicans* Translocation from the Gastrointestinal Tract of Mice by Oral Administration of *Saccharomyces boulardii,*" *The Journal of Infectious Diseases* 168.5 (1993): 1314-318.

188. G. Dalmasso et al., "*Saccharomyces boulardii* Inhibits Inflammatory Bowel Disease by Trapping T Cells in Mesenteric Lymph Nodes," *Gastroenterology* 131.6 (2006): 1812-825.

189. L. Edwards-Ingram et al., "Genotypic and Physiological Characterization of *Saccharomyces boulardii*, the Probiotic Strain of *Saccharomyces cerevisiae,*" *American Society for Microbiology Applied and Environmental Microbiology* 73.8 (2007): 2458-467.

190. M. Guslandi et al., "A Pilot Trial of *Saccharomyces boulardii* in Ulcerative Colitis," *European Journal of Gastroenterology & Hepatology* 15.6 (2003): 697-98.

191. L.V. MacFarland, "Systematic Review and Meta-Analysis of *Saccharomyces boulardii* In Adult Patients," *World Journal of Gastroenterology* 16.18 (2010): 2202-222.

192. S. Moslehi-Jenabian et al., "Beneficial Effects of Probiotic and Food Borne Yeasts on Human Health," *Nutrients* 2.4 (2010): 449-73.

193. A. Murzyn et al., "Capric Acid Secreted by *S. boulardii* Inhibits *C. albicans* Filamentous Growth, Adhesion and Biofilm Formation," *PloS ONE* 5.8 (2010): e12050.

194. Y. Vanderplas et al., "*Saccharomyces boulardii* in Childhood," *European Journal of Pediatrics* 168.3 (2009): 253-65.

195. Iyer, R., S. K. Tomar, T. U. Maheswari, and R. Singh. "*Streptococcus thermophilus* Strains: Multifunctional Lactic Acid Bacteria," *International Dairy Journal* 20.3 (2010): 133-41.

196. M. Elli et al., "Survival of Yogurt Bacteria in the Human Gut," *Applied and Environmental Microbiology* 72.7 (2006): 5113-5117.

197. J.R. Bailey et al., "Identification and Characterisation of an Iron-Responsive Candidate Probiotic," *PloS ONE* 6.10 (2001): e26509.

198. F. Guarner et al., "Should Yoghurt Cultures Be Considered Probiotic?" *British Journal of Nutrition* 93.06 (2005): 783-86.

199. S.E. Gilbreth et al., "Thermophilin 110: A Bacteriocin of *Streptococcus thermophilus* ST110," *Current Microbiology* 51.3 (2005): 175-82.

200. C. Rodríguez, "Therapeutic Effect of *Streptococcus thermophilus* CRL 1190-fermented Milk on Chronic Gastritis," *World Journal of Gastroenterology* 16.13 (2010): 1622-1630.

201. R. Iyer et al., "Dietary Effect of Folate-rich Fermented Milk Produced by *Streptococcus thermophilus* Strains on Hemoglobin Level," *Nutrition* 27.10 (2011): 994-97.

202. S.S. Mousavi et al, "Effects of Medium and Culture Conditions on Folate Production by *Streptococcus thermophilus* BAA-250," *Research in Biotechnology* 4.6 (2013): 21-29.

203. J.P. Burton et al. "Safety Assessment of the Oral Cavity Probiotic *Streptococcus salivarius* K12," *Applied and Environmental Microbiology* 72.4 (2006): 3050–3053.

204. F. Di Pierro et al., "Use of *Streptococcus salivarius* K12 in the Prevention of Streptococcal and Viral Pharyngotonsillitis in Children," *Drug, Healthcare and Patient Safety* 6 (2014): 15-20.

205. W.P. Bowe, "Inhibition of *Propionibacterium acnes* by Bacteriocin-Like Inhibitory Substances (BLIS) Produced by *Streptococcus salivarius*," *Journal of Drugs & Dermatology* 5.9 (2006): 868-70.

206. C. Cosseau et al, "The Commensal *Streptococcus salivarius* K12 Downregulates the Innate Immune Responses of Human Epithelial Cells and Promotes Host-Microbe Homeostasis," *Infection and Immunity* 76.9 (2008): 4163-175.

207. G. Kaci et al., "Anti-Inflammatory Properties of *Streptococcus salivarius*, a Commensal Bacterium of the Oral Cavity and Digestive Tract," *Applied and Environmental Microbiology* 80.3 (2014): 928-34.

About the Author

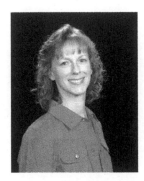 Jo Panyko, B.S., M.N.T. helps people transform their lives by transforming their health! She is a Master Nutrition Therapist with a private nutrition consulting business, Chrysalis Nutrition and Health, LLC. Jo also holds a degree in engineering, created a health-related website, is an accomplished author and is a professional member of the National Association of Nutrition Professionals.

Jo's love of the science behind health and fitness inspired her to create the popular science-based website, *Power of Probiotics*, to teach consumers and healthcare professionals about probiotics. Her passion for health is evident in her website, newsletter, books and various published articles and in her volunteer work as a nutrition educator.

In addition to her insatiable passion for investigating the links between diet, lifestyle, environment and health, Jo enjoys precious time with her husband, children, dogs and friends and is often seen gardening and training for hiking and backpacking adventures. You can contact her at: www.powerofprobiotics.com; on Facebook at PowerOfProbiotics; and on Twitter at PowerOfProbiotx.

Index

Published 1999
Published and distributed in Canada by:
Pallas*Trine Services
P.O. Box 137
Sooke, B.C., Canada
V0S 1N0
Website: www.genio.net/pallas

Canadian Cataloguing in Publication Data

Mills, D. (Donald), date-
    Giant Cedars, White Sands: The Juan de Fuca Marine Trail Guidebook

ISBN 0-9684583-0-0

    1. Hiking--British Columbia--Juan de Fuca Marine Trail--Guidebooks. 2. Juan de Fuca Marine Trail (B.C.)--Guidebooks. I. Title.

GV199.44.C22B7467 1999   917.11'2   C99-900203-1

Cover design by Bobolo & Company, Victoria, B.C.
Edited by Dorothy Jane Mills, a.k.a. Dorothy Z. Seymour
All photographs and maps by the author, Sooke, B.C.
Printed by Digital Direct Printing Ltd. Victoria, B.C.

To the memory of my mother, Audrey Eleanor Mills,
an expert hiker whose affectionate nickname was
"The Mountain Goat"
and who will always be with us in our hearts,
both on and off the trail

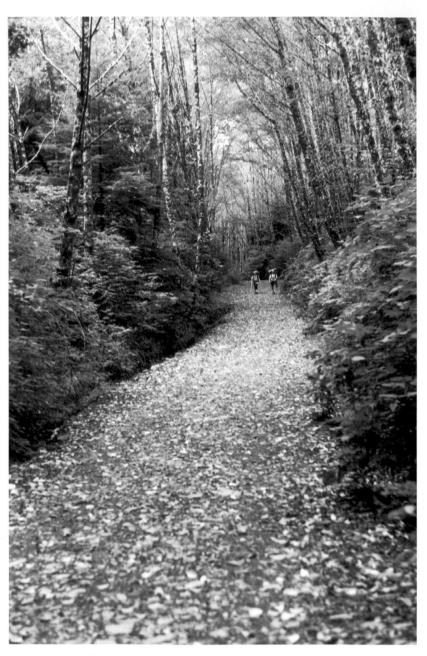

Day Hikers near Botanical Beach

Contents

Acknowledgements

I gratefully acknowledge all those who helped in the preparation of this book, especially my father, Roy Elburt Mills, whose training in hiking and camping gave me a lifelong love for the outdoors. I deeply appreciate the special efforts of my editor, Dorothy Jane Mills, whose expert editing abilities helped forge this book.

A special thanks to my friend, Glenda Primrose, whose help was invaluable in more ways than I can count. Her encouragement and proficient computer abilities were vital in completing this project.

I also appreciate the kind encouragement of Maywell Wickheim and Phoebe Dunbar. I continue to use the information I learned from them.

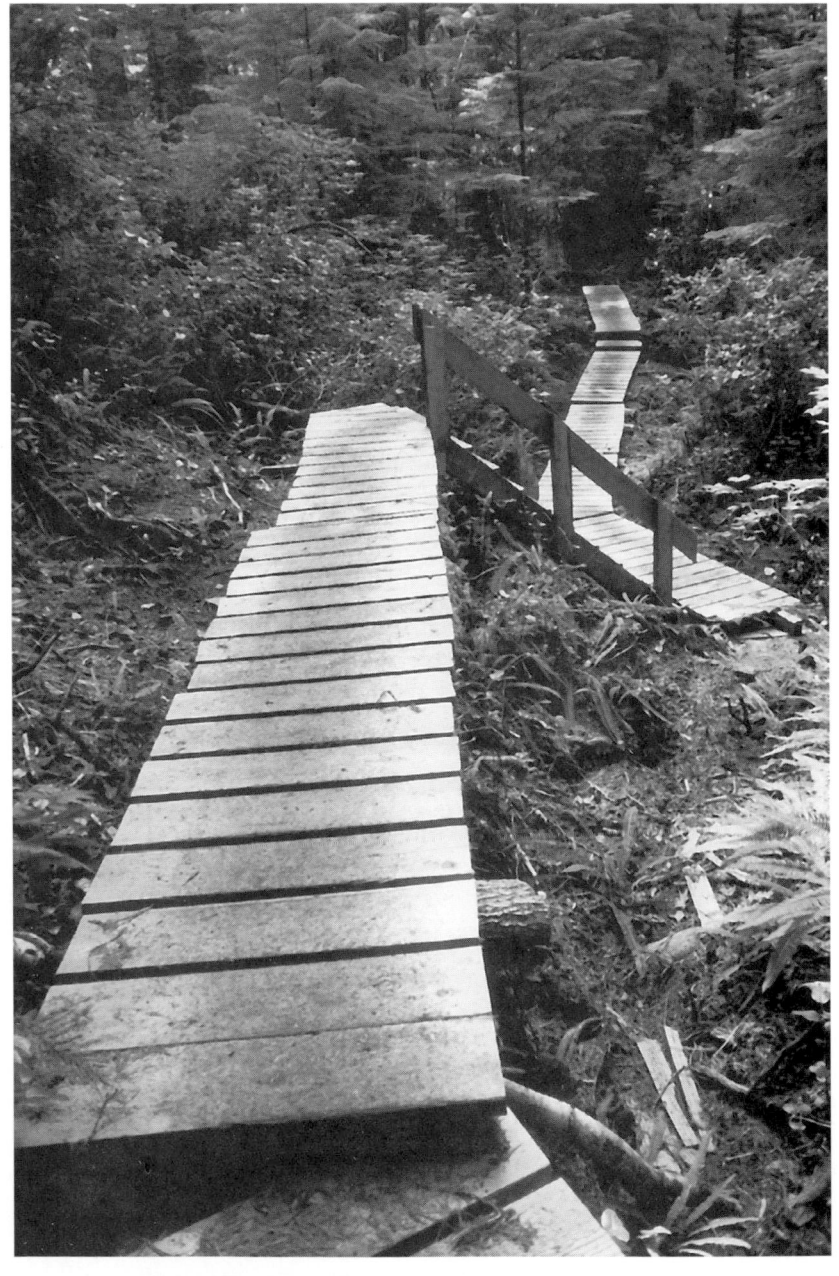

Boardwalks West of Parkinson Creek

Introduction

To the average visitor to British Columbia's Vancouver Island, the southwestern shores are rough and rugged, with few visible signs of activity. A closer look will reveal a wild and beautiful recreational area visited by walking clubs, day hikers, trekkers, kayakers, surfers, weekend campers, photographers, picnickers, bird watchers, and nature lovers. This book is about the new Juan de Fuca Marine Trail, which offers many interesting hiking options. Access points along the Trail allow hikers to enter and exit at several places. Four of these provide pit toilets, parking lots, camp sites, and information boards.

The Juan de Fuca Marine Trail gives hikers the freedom to use the Trail any time. They need not make reservations or pay for trail or ferry permits. The bridges, boardwalks, and suspension bridges are new and very safe. The Trail is forty-seven kilometres long and can be hiked in part, as a day hike, or hiked all at once, in four to six days. Whether you are a novice or an expert hiker, you will want to experience this new and challenging trail.

On the Juan de Fuca Marine Trail, beautiful scenery awaits hikers at nearly every turn. Many spectacular viewpoints overlook the ocean from cliffs, reef shelves, and beaches. Waterfalls and freshwater pools are everywhere on this wilderness hike. The Trail crosses stream after stream as it weaves through the forest of giant Western Hemlock, Red Cedar, and Sitka Spruce. Suddenly it will open up to an ocean view, then just as quickly plunge you back into the forest. The variety of surprises you will encounter makes for real excitement.

This book includes a detailed colour contour map of the Juan de Fuca Marine Trail, information on how to prepare for the trek, and a description of the forty-seven-kilometre trek. You will also find details on interesting trail features, difficult sections, camping spots, tides, day-hiking options, overnight-backpacking trips, and unmarked side trails.

Hikers will quickly see why the Juan de Fuca Marine Trail rates as a world-class adventure hike. I have been on numerous trails, and the Juan de Fuca Marine Trail is one of the best I have ever experienced.

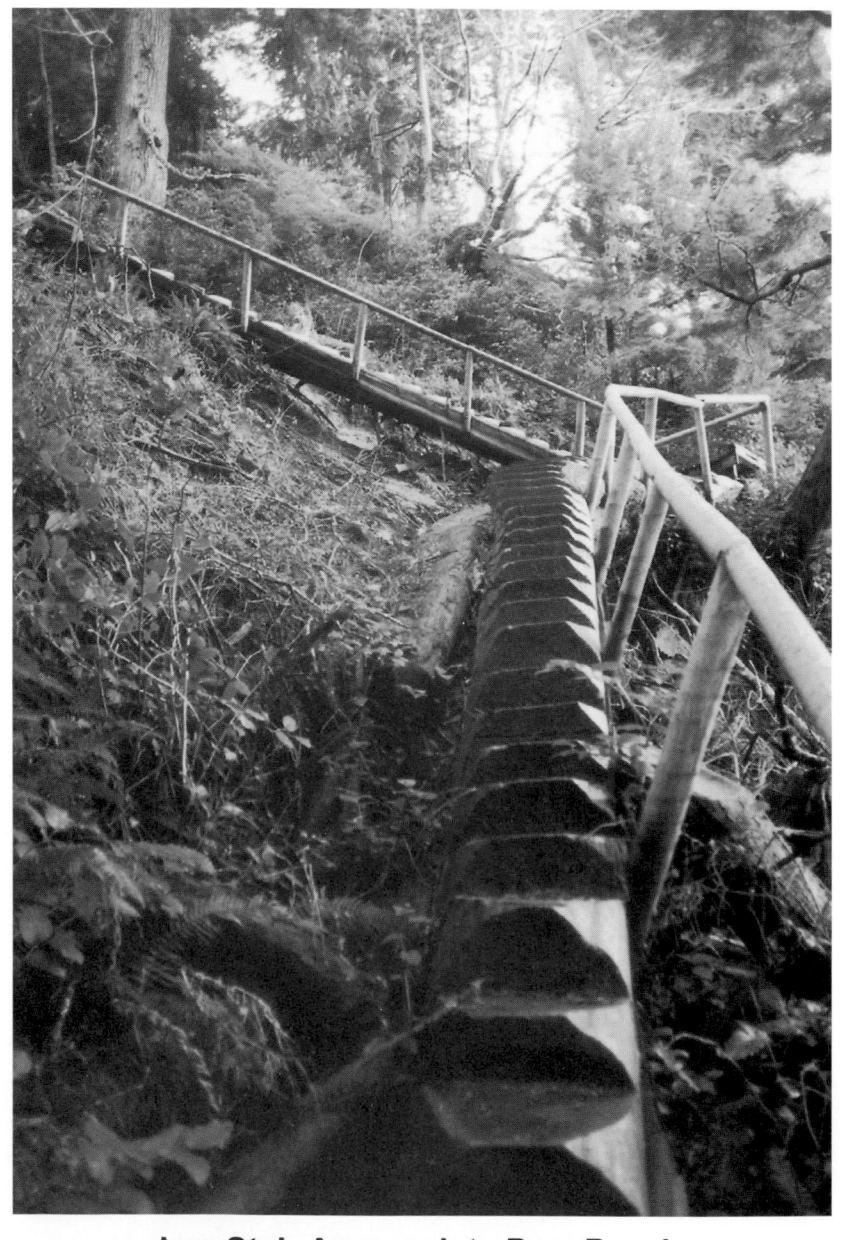

Log Stair Approach to Bear Beach

Chapter 1
Adventure Hiking at Its Best

Welcome to the Juan de Fuca Marine Trail Provincial Park located on the southwestern shores of Vancouver Island. This hiking area stretches along forty-seven kilometres of wild and beautiful rainforest coastline, cradled between Port Renfrew at the west end and Jordan River at the east end. The Coast Mountains directly north of the park supply this forest area with more than forty creeks, which comprise the intricate watershed. To the south, the salt waters of the Juan de Fuca Strait bring ocean storms, waves, and swells to the rocky coastline. The fog banks that often engulf the area enhance the Trail with a magical feeling as hikers make their way through the mists of time.

West Coast rainforests with giant cedars and beautiful white sand beaches are two of the many features one will encounter as the unforgettable experience of hiking this Trail begins to take hold. You will quickly forget all about the city and begin to live the experience of freedom and survival in the forest. You will hear crashing waves and pounding surf along the Trail, where it follows the shoreline cliffs. Caution will be an automatic reaction when you walk across the suspension bridges, which span very deep gorges.

The coastline features vary: rock shelves riddled with tide pools, wave-crafted ocean reefs, towering rocky cliffs, storm-carved caves, boulder beaches, interesting gravel beaches, and soft sandy beaches. If variety constitutes the spice of life, then you have just found the spiciest trail of them all. When walking among the giant trees, you will enjoy the special feeling of the surrounding forest. You will be surprised repeatedly by a new feeling of wonder and awe as you discover the other treasures of the Juan de Fuca Marine Trail.

The flora is diverse along the Trail, with the medium-growth forest the most prevalent, accompanied by ferns, low bushes, old-growth forest trees, mosses, lichens, and horsetails. Different stages of growth in this coastal forest present you with many types of plants. In the areas west of Sombrio, you will get an entirely different feeling as you make your way through the maze of undergrowth. You will never quite see what lies ahead of you, and a flat piece of ground provides a rare but welcome sight. Unique and wonderful geological formations await you here, too. When you come across the thundering rocks three and a half kilometres west of Sombrio River set your pack down and enjoy them for a while. The rock formation on the shoreline funnels waves into a rock tunnel and shoots the water out a blowhole on the other side in a thunderous burst of salt spray.

The Juan de Fuca Marine Trail will give you a first-hand experience of the growth stages of a forest. In some areas, nature has forced a new beginning to the process of establishing the giant trees of the coastal rainforest. Those who want to study the process of forest development can view it all here.

The different sections of the Trail have different conditions for growth and cover for wild animals. Varieties of wild animals live in this ecosystem. As you hike through the forest, keep a lookout for birds, slugs, insects, squirrels, martin, deer, bear, and cougar. Read the trailhead bulletin boards for more information about forest animals.

Walking along the edge of high cliffs or on rocky reef shelves will give you that incredible feeling of being close to nature. Enjoy the breathtaking views from the Trail. Across the Juan de Fuca Strait, the majestic snow-capped Olympic Mountains of Washington State, USA, will add to the feeling of being in a place where time and space seem infinite. Gaze over the waters of the Strait, and you may see grey whales, pods of orca whales, sea lions, seals, and otters.

Tiny marine creatures bustling with life live in the tide pools on Botanical Beach. Botanical Beach Marine Gardens remain protected for all to see and appreciate. Watch the treetops to the east of Botanical Beach; you may see a bald eagle in its natural habitat. Supernatural views will bring you close to nature as you explore the hidden treasures of the forest and beaches.

A hiking trail need not be totally inaccessible to be a good hiking trail. What makes this Trail the best hiking trail on Vancouver Island is its accessibility to everyone. Hikers looking for a true test of their skills will be richly rewarded by the challenges offered on the Juan de Fuca Marine Trail.

This guidebook contains up-to-date information on the Trail. The accompanying map was hand-drawn from information gathered on many recent hikes. Before beginning your hike, review the information in the trip-planning chapter (Chapter 2). You don't want

to spoil a good hike because you forgot something
something you didn't need.

Obtain the appropriate tide guide before your hike, and tak⸜
few minutes to learn how to use your tide tables. Check the
information board at any trailhead to catch any current changes in
policies or other information that may be pertinent. Tide guide
information is usually posted at trailheads on information boards.
Start your hike only after you have this information. You should
arrive at the Trail with your own Tide Guide, which you can print out
directly from the website of this book. **www.genio.net/pallas**

The Juan de Fuca Marine Trail has four main trailheads: China
Beach trailhead, Sombrio Beach trailhead, Creek trailhead, and
Botanical Beach trailhead. Each of these four trailheads provides
parking, information boards, and pit toilets. All the trailheads, with
the exception of Botanical Beach trailhead, allow vehicle camping.
Deposit boxes are available at each of the trailheads for the overnight
(per night) camping fee, presently $5.00 per person. Children 16 years
of age and younger camp on the trail for free when with an adult.
Please read the rules regarding camping and fees on the information
board at any of the trailheads. The fee may change, so be prepared.

HISTORY OF THE TRAIL

The Juan de Fuca Marine Trail has a functional and spiritual
past, linked to the survival of the ancestors of the present-day First
Nations people and the pioneers who first settled the Port Renfrew
area. Logging was the mainstay of the settlers in the area until the
1980s.

Before 1994, the Provincial Government had created small parks
to protect the tide pools, soft sandy beaches, watersheds, pristine
bays, seals, sea lions, and historical native hunting sites. To
commemorate the XVth Commonwealth Games held in 1994 in
Victoria, British Columbia, the provincial and local governments,
along with Western Forest Products Ltd., and Timber West Ltd.,
established the Commonwealth Nature Legacy. This legacy, created
to preserve our living heritage of green space on Southern Vancouver
Island, protects the environment, and provides recreational
opportunities for present and future generations. The Juan de Fuca
Marine Trail Provincial Park, a part of this legacy, opened officially
on April 1, 1996.

government grant funded the work of an
th Team in building the Trail. Because of the
he Trail soon became a world-class trek.

ᴵ JUAN DE FUCA MARINE TRAIL

You caɴ ᵤᵤsily reach the Juan de Fuca Marine Trail from anywhere on the island, the mainland, or even from abroad. Hikers coming to the Island by ferry from Tsawwassen to Swartz Bay, or from abroad by commercial airlines, will arrive on Vancouver Island at the northern end of Saanich Peninsula. Hikers from abroad may want to rent a vehicle. Drive south on the Patricia Bay #17 Highway and exit at McKenzie Avenue. Follow McKenzie Avenue to the #1 Island Highway. Then follow the #1 Island Highway west for three kilometres and exit at the Sooke turnoff onto Highway #14. Highway #14 takes you to Sooke, the Juan de Fuca Marine Trail, and Port Renfrew.

Hikers coming from the City of Victoria will take Douglas Street and travel north out of the city. Douglas Street becomes the #1 Island Highway on leaving Victoria. Take the #1 Island Highway. Exit at the Sooke turnoff, which puts you on Highway #14.

Hikers travelling to the Trail from up-island should take the #1 Highway south to Victoria. Exit from the #1 Island Highway a few kilometres past Goldstream Park at the Sooke Exit #11. Follow the signs at Exit #11, and turn right at the Six Mile Pub, onto #14 Highway.

From the #1 Island Highway exit, follow Highway #14 for thirty kilometres to Sooke. Check your gas at Sooke. The next service station is in Port Renfrew. From Sooke, continue west to the trailhead access of your choice. The four major trailheads are clearly marked with signage along Highway #14. It is approximately thirty-four kilometres from Sooke to the China Beach trailhead and an additional forty-two kilometres to the Botanical Beach trailhead.

Chapter 2
Preparing for Your Trek

Hiking has become one of the most popular recreational pastimes. It is a way to get out and enjoy nature away from the crowded city. To take advantage of the present state of hiking technology, be organized. Take only what you need. Carry the lightest equipment you possibly can when hiking the Juan de Fuca Marine Trail. Many steep hills put your legs to the test. This chapter should help you achieve an efficient backpack that will serve you on this and many other hikes. Remember that a light pack is the supreme goal of every backpacker.

THE BASIC EQUIPMENT

The necessary basics are a backpack, tent, sleeping bag, sleeping pad, stove, and water filter. All these items should be as light as possible.

Backpack: The internal-frame pack is popular with mountain climbers and trekkers traveling with a small amount of weight over difficult terrain. The internal pack fits snugly against your back. Hikers and hunters carrying heavy loads over easy terrain use external-frame packs. Either type of pack is acceptable on the Juan de Fuca Marine Trail.

Distribution of the weight in your pack is important. Light items belong at the bottom of your pack: clothes, foam mattress, and sleeping bag. Heavy items belong at the top of your pack so that the weight rests on your shoulders, not on your lower back.

Use the following table to estimate the maximum weight your full pack should be, including full water bottles.

YOUR BODY WEIGHT	MAXIMUM PACK WEIGHT
45 Kilograms (100 Pounds)	11 Kilograms (25 Pounds)
54 Kilograms (120 Pounds)	14 Kilograms (30 Pounds)
64 Kilograms (140 Pounds)	16 Kilograms (35 Pounds)
73 Kilograms (160 Pounds)	18 Kilograms (40 Pounds)
82 Kilograms (180 Pounds)	20 Kilograms (45 Pounds)
91 Kilograms (200 Pounds)	23 Kilograms (50 Pounds)

Your pack, when full, should not exceed twenty-five percent of your body weight. Carry extra securing pins, tension straps, clips, and a front buckle. A broken strap or buckle can render your backpack inefficient or possibly unusable. Keep the inside of your pack dry by lining it with a plastic garbage bag.

Tent: Decide on the size of tent you will need. The average three-person tent weighs from two to four kilograms (four to eight pounds).

Sleeping Bag: In the summer, if you go backpacking beside the ocean, you will need a sleeping bag rated to at least minus five degrees Celsius (23 degrees Fahrenheit). Strong winds off the ocean can produce wind chills that can make you shiver. Long johns and a thermal top will help you keep your body warmth. Use a hot water bottle to add warmth inside your sleeping bag. Get expert advice before you buy a sleeping bag. Down is excellent, when kept dry. Synthetic fills do the job, and they come at an affordable price.

Sleeping Pad: Foam sleeping pads and thermarests are both popular. Choose the one you like. A sleeping pad will make a big difference in sleeping comfort.

Stove/Fuel: Your stove and fuel should be light. Any of the one-burner stoves on the market are fine. Resist bringing a double-burner Coleman stove. The Juan de Fuca Marine Trail is a coastal rainforest, so do not rely on campfires for cooking. Light your campfires on the beach only below the high-tide mark, and in designated fire pits. Keep fires small and contained.

Remember to pack your food above and away from all fuel in your backpack. Pack the fuel toward the outside of your pack, and near the bottom. If one member of your group carries fuel, another should carry the food. Propane fuels are the safest to carry in a backpack. Consider getting a propane stove if you need to purchase one. Propane fuel is available readily at hardware and camping stores.

Water Filter: All drinking water drawn from streams must be treated or filtered to avoid getting Beaver Fever (Giardia lamblia). A good-quality water filter used properly will filter out the cysts, bacteria, and suspended particles. Another option is to boil your water for three minutes to kill all living organisms in stream water. The third alternative is to put iodine tablets in your water and then let it set fifteen minutes before drinking the water.

16

Get a high-quality water filter so that you can replenish your drinking water fast and efficiently. Avoid drawing drinking water from waterfalls, fast-running water, or stagnant water. Draw water from stream pools, where the particulate matter settles to the bottom. Store drinking water in a wine bladder or water bottle.

SAFETY FIRST

Common sense should prevail when it comes to safety. Hypothermia, Beaver Fever, dehydration, heat exhaustion, blisters, and cuts or fractures are problems you may have to deal with. Be prepared to treat them, and always carry a first aid kit.

Hypothermia: Hypothermia is the Number One cause of medical evacuations on coastal hiking trails. Hypothermia is the profuse loss of heat from the body core to the point where the body cannot regenerate more heat than has been lost. This medical condition can occur during a cold rain or wind when the hiker loses the ability to keep body heat in. ***Hypothermia can be fatal if not controlled swiftly.***

If someone starts shivering, build a fire, and put warmer clothes on the person. Uncontrollable shivering means that person's body has lost the ability to regenerate heat fast enough. Do whatever it takes to get the person warm again. Strip the person, and put him or her in a warmed sleeping bag. A member of your hiking group should strip and join the shivering person to give another source of heat, and to monitor the patient's recovery. Treat this as a serious medical emergency. When the patient is warm again, administer a hot meal and lots of warm liquids.

Prevention is better than the cure. Prevent severe heat loss by wearing the appropriate clothing. When it rains, wear proper rain gear. Wear a hat to help prevent heat loss from the head. After a day of hiking, take off wet shorts or T-shirt and put on warm, dry clothes. Long johns, fleece jacket, thermal socks, hat, and tea or soup will help you keep warm when the sun goes down.

Beaver Fever: Beaver and other wild animals' feces often contain Giardia lamblia, a type of intestinal cyst. When animal droppings fall into water, the cysts, when present, become waterborne. The cysts are capable of causing a very serious illness referred to as Beaver Fever. If a human ingests the Giardia lamblia cyst, the resulting infection will cause acute diarrhea and nausea, and it can take years to expel from the body tissue. Prevent this parasite from infecting you by filtering or treating all your drinking water. Before drinking water from any creek or river, boil the water, treat it with iodine tablets, or use a very good-quality water filter. Don't let Beaver Fever happen to you.

Dehydration: Drink lots of water before, during, and after hiking. On a six-hour hike, keep your water bottle handy, and drink a minimum of four or five litres of water. If you become thirsty, you are experiencing a mild dehydration A sure sign of dehydration is a dry mouth. Another sign is dark yellow urine. Dehydration will result in decreased endurance and increased fatigue. Heavy perspiration can lead to rapid fluid loss. Alcohol and caffeine can dehydrate you as well.

Heat Exhaustion: Dehydration and heat exhaustion usually occur together, but not always. Carry an umbrella or wear a hat when hiking in the hot sun for extended periods (for example, on Bear Beach). If you succumb to heat exhaustion, you will become tired, dizzy, and lethargic. Prevention includes avoiding hiking for long periods in the hot sun and drinking plenty of water.

Blisters: Blisters can be very painful, so make it your priority to prevent them. Keep your pack weight below twenty-five percent of your body weight. Wear properly fitting backpacking boots and wear two pairs of socks. Inner socks made of polypropylene draw moisture away from the feet and keep them dry. The outer wool socks will adsorb moisture and help keep the feet dry and warm. The two layers of socks also prevent friction between the boot and the foot. In addition, protect your boots with a water-repellent boot sealer. Wear new boots every day at home for at least a week before wearing them on the trail.

Cuts and Fractures: If you incur a fracture on the trail and can't continue hiking, send for help. Dress small cuts and scrapes with rubbing alcohol, iodine, antibacterial cream, and a sterile bandage or wrap. If you trip over a log, your hands usually go out in front of you to break the fall. Wear biking gloves to protect the palms of your hands from cuts and slivers.

First-Aid Kit: Keep your first-aid kit light and small. Choose small containers, or repackage some items into smaller containers. Rubbing alcohol usually comes in 100-ml containers. You need only bring 10 ml or less in a tiny bottle. Put your first-aid pouch into a sealed baggie to keep it dry. First-aid kits should include the following items:

Emergency Flare (signal)
Emergency Space Blanket (for hypothermia victims)
Tweezers (remove slivers)
Small Scissors (many uses)
Nail Clippers (keep toe nails short, and cut thread)
Suture Needles (stitch up cuts and gashes)
Suture Thread (four feet is enough)
Pain Killers (for an emergency)
Bandages (for cuts and scrapes)
Gauze (one roll will do)
Lighter (sterilize needles)
Duct Tape (for splints, repairs, etc.)
Iodine (stops bleeding)
Antiseptic Towelettes or cream (disinfects the wound)
Antibiotic Cream (stops infection)
Bee Sting Kit (for wasp and bee stings)
Tiger Balm (for sore muscles)
Tensor Bandage (for sore knees)
Corn Pads (put over blister to keep pressure off it)
Second Skin (soft, moistened blister padding)
Moleskin (put over Second Skin)
Aspirin (stops a wound from swelling)
Swiss Army Knife (multiple uses)
Matches (waterproof)

Getting Help: In an emergency, use the closest exit to reach Highway #14 to go for help. Know the exact location of the victim. Phone 911. The Sooke Search and Rescue Volunteer Team operating out of Sooke, B.C. stays on 24-hour emergency standby to rescue injured, lost, and missing hikers. Carrying a long-range analog-type cell phone is a good idea. In recent years, cell phones have helped save several hikers' lives.

CLOTHING

The basic hiking clothes consist of good boots, rain gear, camp clothes, hiking clothes, socks, and gaiters.

Hiking Boots: The most important piece of clothing you have is your hiking boots. Choose boots with good ankle support. You do not need mountaineer's boots. Instead, ask at a reputable outdoor store for lightweight backpacking boots.

Protect leather boots with a waterproof leather protector if you want your boots to last a long time, and keep your feet dry and blister-free. Purchase a good-quality boot protector paste and apply it to your boots before, during, and after every hike. Boot protector is necessary for your leather boots if rain is in the forecast.

Rain Gear: Bring a water-resistant, seam-sealed rain jacket with a hood. Rain pants are good to have in a major downpour, as is an umbrella. An umbrella is an item I always bring. It can supply shade when the sun is hot, or scare off wild animals by giving the illusion that you are bigger than you actually are when the umbrella is open.

Camp Clothes: Light cotton or wind pants, a cotton shirt, and thermal underwear should keep you warm in camp. A fleece top is light and warm and should be all you need to keep warm in the cool evenings, but if you are still cold, put the rain jacket on. Bring clothes that serve more than one purpose. Use thermal underwear as pajamas if you are cold when inside your sleeping bag.

Fill watertight containers and wine bladders with hot water and place in your sleeping bag for extra warmth. Bring camp shoes to wear after the day's hike to give your hiking boots a chance to air out. When you are at a campsite and not carrying a pack, you can wear sandals, sneakers, reef boots, or any other light shoes. Many hikers prefer reef boots because you can get them wet and still keep your feet warm. Bring twelve metres of three-millimeter cord to use as a clothesline for drying out wet socks or T-shirts.

Note: The only clothing items you will need more than one of are: underwear, T-shirts, liner socks, and wool outer socks. Tightly wrap spare clothing in clear cling wrap, and then put your spare clothes in smaller stuff-sacks.

Hiking Clothes: The ideal hiking attire is a T-shirt, hiking shorts, and a cotton hiking shirt. When you first start out on a day's hike, you may want to bundle up to keep warm. You will quickly learn that your body temperature will rise because of exertion. As the day gets warmer, you will most certainly become warmer as you continue to hike. Your body usually cools down when you stop. To prevent a chill, wear the shirt when you stop for a rest, and tie it to the top of your pack while you are hiking.

Socks: Wearing the proper socks is very important. Hiking with the wrong socks may give you blisters. You should wear two pairs of socks. The inner socks should be of light polypropylene. This material draws moisture away from your feet. Moist feet are more prone to blisters than dry feet.

The outer pair of socks should be made of slightly heavier wool to hold the moisture away from your feet. The boot will rub against the outer sock, but the inner sock keeps the rubbing away from your foot, thus preventing blisters. Keeping your socks and feet dry and clean, and carrying a light pack, will help prevent blisters.

Gore-Tex waterproof socks are expensive but will keep your feet dry in a downpour. If you have a pair, don't leave home without them.

Gaiters: When hiking in the woods or on a sandy beach, you kick up particles of dust or grains of sand. To prevent dust or sand from entering between your socks and the inner surface of your boots, wear a pair of gaiters. Most varieties of gaiters rise to the top of the shin, just below the knee, and completely cover the laces and heel of the boot. Protection against insects and low, sharp branches adds to the value of wearing gaiters. An old pair of socks with the soles cut out makes an effective substitute for gaiters.

PERSONAL

The following are some of the personal items you will want to bring. Many of these items are optional, but if your pack weight allows, having them with you will make your hike a lot more pleasant. Choose items that are light and small.

Gloves: Protect the palms of your hands with a pair of bicycle gloves. You will save your hands from slivers, scrapes, and maybe even burns. Wear light work gloves when using the camp stove or collecting driftwood.

Utensils: Bring a small cooking pot, a water bottle, a wine bladder for filtered drinking water, a thermal cup, and a small spoon.

Toiletries: Bring biodegradable soap, a small towel, a facecloth, toilet paper, dental floss, a toothbrush, a small tube of toothpaste, a hairbrush, and sunscreen. Do not bathe or wash in fresh water sources. Take sponge baths, or bring a portable shower.

The Little Necessary Things: Bring a small flashlight (one per tent), a whistle or bells, boot wax, an extra pair of bootlaces, an umbrella (this is a coastal rainforest), a wristwatch (to use the tide tables), and a small camera. You may also want to bring a small waist pack for carrying daily items.

Sewing Kit: Put the following items in a labeled film cartridge: three large-eyed needles, a few metres of heavy thread, four safety pins, and some buttons.

FOOD

Choose light, dehydrated foods that are fast to prepare. Keep up your strength and energy levels by eating lots of snacks on the trail. While at a campsite, protect your food in a pack from animals, rain, and dew. At night hoist all food at least four metres up a tree. Bring twelve metres of five-millimeter cord for hanging food away from wild animals at night. Hang the food at least two metres away from the tree trunk. Bears, cougars, squirrels, martins, chipmunks, mice, birds, and many other forest animals can smell your food and other goodies from miles away. Never keep food in your tent.

Breakfast: Start your day with nutritious cereals, powdered milk, nuts, dried fruit, and sweetener.

Lunch: A quick lunch can be made with cheese, crackers, bagels, canned paté, pepper sausage, soup mix, hot chocolate, and energy drinks.

On a rainy day, make your luncheon soup right after you have cooked your breakfast. If you are boiling water at breakfast, then boil some extra water for soup that you will eat at lunchtime. Put the soup in a wide-mouth water bottle, and wrap it in your towel or shirt to keep it warm. This advance preparation saves you from unpacking stoves and pots while you are on the trail. When you need something warm and nutritious to eat, your lunch will be ready.

Snacks: Munch on energy bars, trail mix, dried fruit, and other high-energy snacks.

Dinner: Choose light foods like rice or instant potatoes, bagels, dried meat or fish, tea, vitamins, soup, and dried vegetables.

Do not wash dishes in fresh water sources. Avoid leaving any trace of your visit in this park. Pack out all cans, plastics, cigarette butts, paper, and any other items that are not completely and quickly biodegradable. If in doubt, pack it out.

TIDES, BEACHES, AND WAVES

Tides: Hikers must be able to read a tide guide before hiking this Trail because certain points on the trail are under water when the tides are high. Take the time to learn this easy skill. ***When hiking, be sure to carry a current tide guide for the Sooke area.*** In order to use the tide guide, you will also need a watch.

Know how to use your tide guide to help you plan an enjoyable hike. Use the tide tables to find the extreme low tides for the year. On days when the tide is below 1.2 metres, you may want to visit the tide pools at Botanical Beach and other choice spots. Plan your hike accordingly.

Beaches: Several high-tide cutoffs along the Trail may present a problem if you arrive at high tide. Use the tide tables to help you time your hike to arrive at these locations at low tide. ***Special Note:*** High-tide cutoff #3 at Chin Beach West extends from Km. 21.5 to Km. 22.2 and stays impassible most of the time. It is passable only at full- and new-moon low tides below one metre. Use the forest route most of the time. The rocky point at Km. 21.5 becomes impassable at tides above 2.75 metres. A beach marker buoy points westbound hikers to use the main forest route.

Beach marker buoys are about the size of basketballs, are red in color, and placed high up in trees very close to where the Trail meets the beach. Look for these buoys while hiking on the beaches to locate where the Trail continues back into the forest.

Waves: Rogue waves can sweep a hiker off a rock shelf without warning, so keep your eye on incoming waves when on a beach or reef shelf beside the ocean. Take note that the seventh wave is usually larger than the preceding six waves. Watch the ocean waves and discover this phenomena for yourself.

BEGINNING YOUR HIKE

Hikers who are in tune with their surroundings will feel at home in the forest. Remember the time-honored Boy Scout motto, "Be Prepared." It could save your life or someone else's. Use common sense in the forest. Travel light, and have a great hike.

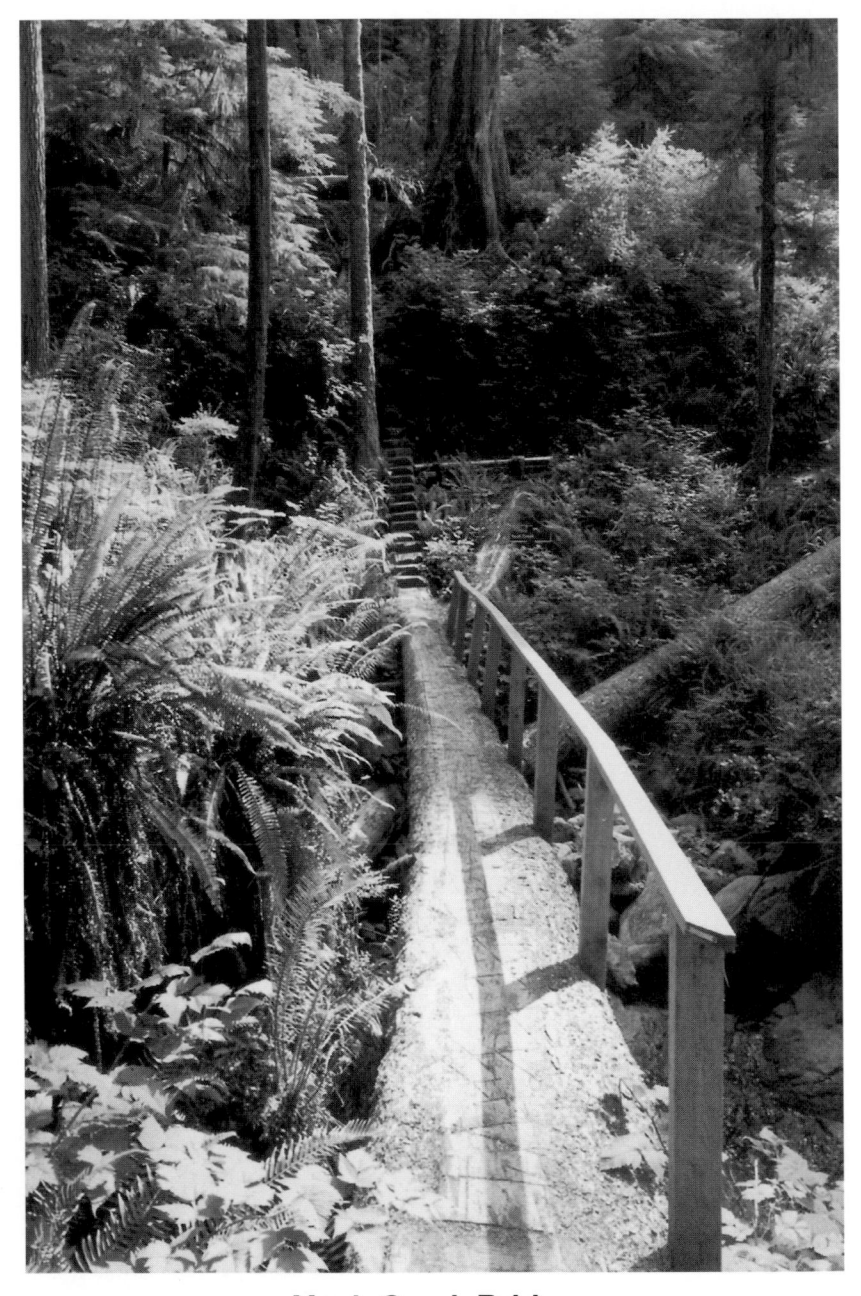

Yauh Creek Bridge

Chapter 3
Forty-seven Kilometres of
Wilderness Trekking

The Juan de Fuca Marine Trail stretches forty-seven kilometres from China Beach trailhead to Botanical Beach trailhead. The Trail remains open to hikers all year round. To give trekkers a guide for organizing their hike, I have divided the trek into five sections. Each section covers approximately ten kilometres, which constitutes a reasonable distance to hike each day on this trail. If you are an experienced trekker, you may want to hike more than one section at once, but keep in mind what lies ahead. Use only designated camping spots.

Having arrived at the Juan de Fuca Marine Trail trailhead at China Beach or Botanical Beach, you will want to orient yourself to the Trail. Those hikers starting their trek from Botanical Beach can follow the sections described here in reverse order.

You will find two parking lots located at the China Beach trailhead. The lower parking lot accesses only China Beach while the upper parking lot serves the Juan de Fuca Marine Trail trailhead. The lower parking lot is for day use only. You may car camp in the upper parking lot. Be sure to check the information boards for any Trail news, such as recent bear or cougar sightings, and for directions on what to do in case of a bear or cougar encounter.

Print the tide tables from the book website (p.94), or copy down the appropriate tide tables from the information board, or buy tide tables from Eagle-Eye store in Sooke. High-tide beach cutoff areas may delay your hike if you arrive at the high tide for that day. Bring a wristwatch so you can use your tide tables, and keep in mind that large ocean swells tend to raise the height of the ocean water level.

Camping fees apply on the Trail and at the trailhead parking lots. Hikers may car-camp at the upper parking lot at China Beach, at Sombrio Beach parking lot, and at Parkinson Creek parking lot. Read the instructions before depositing your fee into the vault. Deposit boxes are available at each of the trailheads for the overnight backcountry (per night) camping fee, presently $5.00 per person. Children 16 years old and under camp for free. You can check on any

25

changes in the camping fee by contacting BC Parks in Victoria by phone: 1-250-391-2300, e-mail: *wwwmail@pubaffair.env.gov.bc.ca* , or by fax: 1-250-478-9211.

Look after all the last-minute preparations, and get yourself ready to set out on your hike. Nothing compares to that moment when you slip into your pack harness and get ready to take those first steps of your trek. Twenty minutes after commencing your hike, your body will warm up dramatically. I recommend wearing hiking shorts and a T-shirt from the outset so that you need not change clothes along the Trail. Wear gaiters and two pair of socks to help prevent blisters.

As you hike, you will perspire. Replace this loss of water from your body by drinking water often. To prevent dehydration, try to drink a minimum of three to four litres of water every day while hiking.

Now that you're all prepared for your hike, you're ready to start. Here's a detailed description of the Trail, divided into five sections:

> A. China Beach to Bear Beach
>
> B. Bear Beach to Chin Beach
>
> C. Chin Beach to Sombrio Beach
>
> D. Sombrio Beach to Parkinson Creek
>
> E. Parkinson Creek to Botanical Beach

Sections A and B will each take a day to hike. Most hikers can complete sections C, D, and E in three days. Advanced hikers may decide to complete sections C, D, and E in two days.

Do not hike beyond your limits. Try to plan where you will camp and how far you will hike in a day. You may want to review the hidden treasures detailed in Chapter 6 to plan extra time for exploring.

A. CHINA BEACH TRAILHEAD TO BEAR BEACH

Distance:	10.5 kilometres (Km. 0 to Km. 10.5)
Difficulty Rating:	intermediate
Average Hiking Time:	from 5 to 7 hours
Description of Trail:	open forest and beach hiking
Beach Camping:	at Km. 2.5, Km. 8.6, and from Km. 9.4 to Km. 10.5
High-tide Beach Cutoff:	at Km. 8.7 on Bear Beach

The first two kilometres of your hike start you off with an easy jaunt through the forest over roots, around stumps, and beside fallen trees. A suspension bridge crosses **Pete Wolf Creek** one kilometre from the trailhead.

As you approach **Mystic Beach (Km. 2.2)**, forty minutes into your hike, the sound of the surf gets louder. The steep trail, which descends to the beach, can often be muddy and slippery. As you walk from the Trail to the beach, you will see an information board by the Trail and a red marker ball hanging in a tree overhead. Marker balls hang over the trail at the point where the Trail meets the beach to guide you in finding the Trail from the beach.

If you want to see all of Mystic Beach, hike to the east end below the cliffs. As you pass a little waterfall coming down from the cliff above, you can walk on hard-packed white sand when the tide is low. As you walk along Mystic Beach, make a note of the great camping spots on the western half of the beach. The soft white sand attracts many weekend campers to this beach. *See a picture of Mystic Beach on the colour contour map.*

At the west end of Mystic Beach, near **McVicar Creek (Km. 2.6)**, a marker ball and trail sign point to where the Trail continues westward into the forest. At low tide, explore the large rock arch at the extreme west end of Mystic Beach, just one of the many geological wonders along the trail. As you leave Mystic Beach, the Trail climbs into the forest and follows along the bluff.

At Km. 3.3, an open-faced cliff reveals an unobstructed panoramic ocean view, one of the few such views on this section of the Trail. From these cliffs, you might even spot a whale. The Trail soon crosses over **Pat Philip Creek (Km. 3.6)** on a sturdy wooden bridge. Here many hikers empty their bottles of city water and filter fresh stream water from the pools that lie five metres below the bridge. The next few kilometres bring excellent forest hiking, high cliffs, and deep creek beds. A wooden bridge traverses **Bent Creek (Km. 5.0)**. Many pools and a wide streambed invite exploring. Include exploring in your hike in order to give your back a rest from carrying that heavy pack. After your hike, you will remember exploring more vividly than you will remember hiking along the Trail with a pack on your back. Another viewpoint at Km. 5.5 rises forty metres above the beach. On a clear day, you'll be able to enjoy views of the Olympic Mountains. Watch for ships and whales from this viewpoint.

The wooden bridge at **Fatt Creek (Km. 6.1)** spans steep embankments and the fast-flowing water in the creek bed below. Canteen water could be a bit tricky to obtain here, so be careful.

Just past **Fatt Creek at Km. 6.2**, the Trail incorporates a big fallen tree that crosses an old creek bed. Notches in the tree help you keep your footing when the log becomes wet from rain or fog. The log lies only a few metres above the creek bed, so this crossing will not intimidate hikers who fear heights.

A sturdy wooden bridge crosses **Ivanhoe Creek (Km. 7.5)**, where pools, a fresh-water stream, and the creek bed invite exploration. The creek bed lies nearly seven metres below the bridge.

As you make the approach to Bear Beach, you will hear the surf crashing on the beach below. Just after Km. 8.0, enjoy the descent to Bear Beach on wooden stairs carved into a tree trunk. The stairs accommodate only one hiker at a time, so please give the right of way to hikers coming up the stairs. A thick cable keeps the stairs secured in place. This dramatic descent to Bear Beach affords spectacular views of the surrounding area. Where the Trail meets the beach, you will find the beach marker ball hanging overhead in a tree and the information board posted with maps and bear/cougar information.

Bear Beach (Km. 8.2 to 10.5) stretches for three kilometres from end to end. Four creeks and three camping areas make this a perfect spot to spend the night. Keep your campsite close to a source of fresh water so that you can easily carry water for cooking and washing dishes. If you have lots of time, you can explore the creek beds, or beachcomb, or even watch for whales. The lack of designated camping between Bear Beach and Chin Beach makes camping on Bear Beach a certainty. At the extreme east end of Bear Beach, you may want to explore the rock arch under the cliff at low tide. If you arrive here at high tide, you will have to save this little walk for another time.

Continue west on Bear Beach to **Rosemond Creek (Km. 8.6)**. Heavy rains may render the creek swollen. Use fallen logs to get across. If the high tide blocks the Trail at the cliff just beyond Rosemond Creek, you may want to stop for lunch or pitch the tent rather than getting your hiking boots wet.

You will find great campsites on both sides of Rosemond Creek. You can use the pit toilets on the west side of the creek. If you want to see deep pools and little falls and hear the babbling sounds of the creek water, go exploring up the creek bed. Make your way past the fallen tree across the creek, and you will be in your own private little ecosystem. Filter your fresh water from the creek pools.

The **high-tide beach cutoff** immediately west of Rosemond Creek becomes impassable when the tide rises above three metres. Large waves crashing on the beach may even render the cutoff impassible at lower tides. If you can see solid ground, the cutoff remains passable. *See the picture (looking west) of this cutoff area at low tide on the colour contour map.*

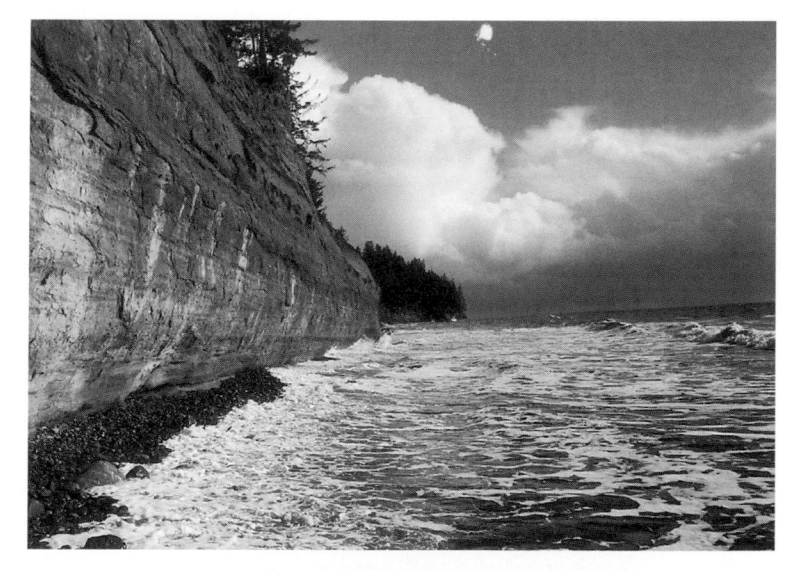

Bear Beach Cutoff at High Tide
(Looking East)

29

One kilometre west of Rosemond Creek you will discover Clinch Creek. Pit toilets and campsites are located on either side of the creek. An unmarked side trail just 35 paces east of the mouth of Clinch Creek (Km. 9.6) leads up to Highway #14. *See Chapter 5 for a complete description of this side trail and other side trails located along the Juan de Fuca Marine Trail.*

Watch for the old rusted iron artifacts from a shipwreck lying on the beach west of Clinch Creek at Km. 10. The sandy beach and camping spots on the point reveal a panoramic view of the Juan de Fuca Strait. More cozy campsites, pit toilets, and an information board await discovery just around the point.

Near **Ledingham Creek (Km. 10.5)** find more great campsites blessed with a perfect view of Mushroom Rock, a geological structure now called Rock-on-a-Pillar. The mushroom-shaped rock, crafted by many years of tide and wave action, projects from the inter-tidal zone on this picturesque part of Bear Beach.

At the extreme west end of Bear Beach, just beyond all the signs, the beach trail marker ball leads hikers back to the forest trail at Ledingham Creek. The Trail begins directly beside the mouth of the creek. What lies ahead? I hope you had a good rest last night!

B.   BEAR BEACH TO CHIN BEACH

Distance:	10.5 kilometres (Km. 10.5 to Km. 21)
Difficulty Rating:	most difficult
Average Hiking Time:	from 5 to 8 hours
Description of Trail:	forest on hilly terrain, and beach hiking
Beach Camping:	from Km. 9.5 to Km. 10.5, and at Km. 21
High-tide Beach Cutoff:	at Km. 20.5

The next eleven kilometres, between Bear Beach and Chin Beach, epitomize the very best of forest hiking. Many old-growth trees stand in the forest, and some estimates put the age of the more mature trees at nearly a thousand years. The steep slopes on this section of the Trail may constitute a challenge to some hikers, but this part remains my favorite section. Use the creeks, beaches, and trail turns to keep yourself oriented.

The next two kilometres past **Ledingham Creek (Km. 10.5)** let you experience steep and grueling hills that punish your legs and your ego. Follow the Trail from the creek mouth up a very steep climb to the top of the hill. The eighty-metre climb tests your legs all the way up and during your descent to the next creek bed. From this unnamed creek, spanned by a solid wooden bridge, you will again climb up to the top of the next hill and then down again. Take a rest at **Hoard Creek (Km. 12),** a pause you will surely welcome at the bottom of the second hill. *Remember to drink plenty of water on today's hike.*

While at Hoard Creek enjoy the view of the ocean, a secluded little beach, and a streambed full of freshwater pools. A clearing by the bridge gives you a place to set down your pack for a rest. The clear babbling creek water courses through beautiful pools in the streambed. Tiny trout have claimed a few pools as their home.

A short trail in front of the bridge leads down to a small beach and to the streambed. The high tides usually flood the beach, so do not set up your tent on this beach. Should an emergency arise, the clearing beside the bridge would make a good place to put up your tent for the night. Hoard Creek gives you an opportunity to replenish your water bottles. Explore up the creek bed, and give yourself a well-deserved rest from your pack.

Expect a long, steady climb uphill from Hoard Creek to an old logging road. As you get close to the old road, the Trail levels out. Near Km. 13, the road and Trail run adjacent to each other for several metres. Stay on the Trail. Hikers may access Highway #14 via the old logging road in an emergency. *See Chapter 5 for a complete description of this side trail and other side trails located along the Trail.*

From Km. 13, the Trail follows the bluff around to a ridge, where it takes a gradual descent to **Newmarch Creek (Km. 14)**. You will encounter some deep mud holes along the way. Newmarch Creek bridge consists of two planks. Not very elaborate, but it gets you across. Many small bathtub-sized pools of water in the creek bed make Newmarch Creek another fine spot to fill your canteen. These pools give the creek bed the appearance of the face of a giant space creature. The wide creek bed invites exploration upstream for a short distance.

The Trail climbs up to the next ridge and follows the bluff, offering views of the ocean. While hiking, you will see ferns and large trees, and you'll hear ocean waves crashing on the beaches and rocky shore below. The soft loam trail feels like a large rubber mat below your feet, cushioning every step as you hike along through the forest.

For the next few kilometres, the Trail follows the bluff. Before arriving at Chin Beach, you will descend several times to deep creek beds and climb back up to the bluff. During light rain or heavy fog, the Trail, which lies under the forest canopy, stays relatively dry. This section of the Trail remains my favorite terrain for day hikes. Draw water for drinking from the creek pools at Km. 17. Use a rope and a pot to dip the water from the three-metre-deep creek bed.

The next kilometre brings more excellent hiking. The Trail along the cliff towers fifty metres above the ocean surf. **Lines Creek (Km. 18.7)**, crossed by a log bridge, greets the ocean with a ten-metre drop over a rock ledge straight down to the beach. Even after an extensive search along this section, I found no way to climb down to the beach below. If you need to stretch your back without your pack on, explore up Lines Creek.

From Lines Creek, the Trail weaves through the old-growth forest, down a few creek beds, across two solid bridges, then past waterfalls, pools, and a few more inaccessible, secluded beaches. Switchbacks up to Km. 20 bring you to the final approach to **Chin Beach (Km. 20.5)**.

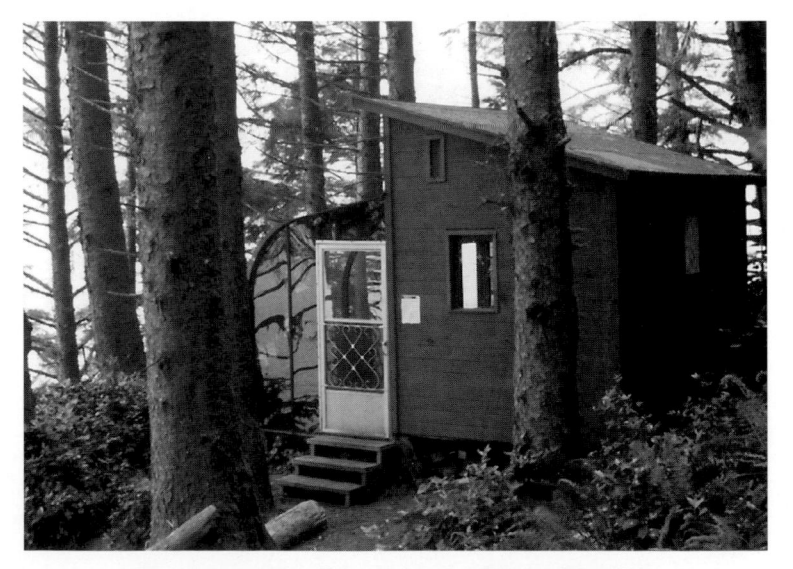

Emergency Shelter At Chin Beach

On the bluff at the east end of Chin Beach, an Emergency Shelter equipped with a sunroom and two small lofts welcomes you. *If you visit this shelter, please sign the guest book.* If you've hiked all day in the rain, you may decide to stay in the shelter overnight and dry out. From the cabin, you will descend the steep slope to the reef shelf below. If ocean waves prevent you from accessing the beach at the reef shelf high-tide cutoff, wait in the cabin.

At the centre of Chin Beach, the camping area becomes apparent, because hikers have erected numerous driftwood fences on the beach to block the wind at individual campsites. *When you break camp, please help to keep the beach looking natural by scattering your firepit rocks and driftwood windbreaks.* At Km. 21, use the small stream as your freshwater source.

To view some giant cedar trees, follow the hidden side trail, located behind the campsite at Km. 21. *See the map and information in Chapter 5: Unmarked Side Trail #4 - Chin Beach at Km. 21.*

C. CHIN BEACH TO SOMBRIO BEACH

Distance:	8.0 kilometres (Km. 21 to Km. 29)
Difficulty Rating:	difficult
Average Hiking Time:	from 4 to 6 hours
Description of Trail:	forest, beach, old gravel road
Beach Camping:	at Km. 21, and from Km. 27.5 to Km. 29
High-tide Beach Cutoff:	from Km. 21.3 to 22.1, and at Km. 27.8 Note: The high-tide beach cutoff on Chin Beach extending from Km. 21.3 to Km. 22.1 remains impassible most of the time. This beach area becomes passable only at extreme full- and new-moon low tides. In general, use the forest route.

Eight kilometres full of interesting places to explore characterize the wilderness between Chin Beach and Sombrio Beach. Special attractions include the gorge at Loss Creek, the sea lion caves, hidden waterfalls, and Sombrio Beach. Trekkers may camp on Sombrio Beach or continue on to Little Kuitsche Creek, where forest camping prevails.

From the camp area on **Chin Beach (Km. 21)**, continue west along the beach to the rocky **high-tide cutoff** point at Km. 21.3. The beach cutoff between Km. 21.3 and 22.1 remains under water most of the time. Waves make this area of the beach very dangerous, even when the tide falls below one metre. **This entire cut-off area becomes passable only at extreme full- and new-moon tides. At all other times use the forest trail.**

Look for the marker ball hanging in the tree at the rocky point of the high-tide cutoff (Km. 21.3). Follow the Trail up into the forest and look for the information board at the stream, located 50 metres west of Km. 22. The shallow stream and the information board (in the forest) mark the west end of Chin Beach. If you wish to explore the west end of the beach, walk on the west side of the streambed where a marker buoy shows the way to a steep access point.

Continue hiking west on the forest trail. Prepare yourself for a steep climb to the top of the hill. At the top, you can sit down and rest, or follow the Trail all the way down to the bottom of the next creekbed. Large trees, ferns, and low bushes comprise much of the forest foliage. A soft loam trail on the forest floor makes for good footing. A rest area greets you immediately before **Loss Creek (Km. 23.8)**. If your legs cramp up, give them a long rest.

Crossing the Loss Creek suspension bridge is fun, but you may get butterflies in your stomach from looking down at the creek below. West of Loss Creek, the Trail climbs pleasantly up into the woods and up the hill toward the old logging road. Just five minutes past Loss Creek, the marker for Km. 24 appears, and the uphill walk to the old logging road begins. Before arriving at the road, you will encounter a section of thick forest that blocks out a lot of sunlight because of a dense canopy overhead.

The old logging road greets you with trail-direction signs and a rusted cable strewn on the road. At this point, a hidden side trail leads to the sea lion observation rocks. *See Chapter 6: Hidden Treasures, #6 - Gorge, Sea Lion Caves and Reef Shelf (at Km. 25)*.

For the next kilometre, enjoy the flat surface of the old logging road. This road is one of the few level places on the Trail. The end of the road at Km. 26 marks the beginning of the descent on a steep ridge to **Sombrio Viewpoint (Km. 26.5)**.

Follow the cliff around to Km. 27 to view the waterfall at the east end of Sombrio Beach. Keep your footing while following this dangerously slippery cliff face. A long tree trunk with stairs carved into it welcomes you with a perfect view of Sombrio Beach, and at the end of the tree staircase, a view of the waterfall. A wooden bridge crosses the creek at the east end of Sombrio Beach. You will pass refreshing pools on the ledge. Farther up this creekbed, explore and discover more pretty falls and pools.

After another ten minutes of forest hiking, the final approach to **Sombrio Beach (Km. 27)** appears before your eyes. Here you will find a Trail information board, plenty of campsites, and pit toilets close by. A red marker ball hangs in a tree above the trail leading to the beach.

When you arrive at the beach, climb over the long fallen tree jutting out over the surf. Just west of the tree, a stream flows out of the woods. Follow the streambed as far as you can for a view of the hidden ten-metre-high waterfall. By stepping on logs in the stream, you can stand right beside the falls and see the hidden pool. *Wear reef boots or sandals, if you brought a pair. I generally bring reef boots on my hikes to use as camp shoes and to explore up streams.* Immediately east of the little stream, several camping spots come into view on the bank above the beach.

A short distance down the beach, and directly in front of your view at Km. 27.8, looms a **high-tide cutoff**. At low tide, you can hike around this first point and past the little caves in the rock. If the tide rises above three metres, it will stop you from proceeding any farther. Plan to arrive here at the low tide of the day, because no alternate route exists.

At Sombrio Beach, you'll discover the best campsites on the entire Trail. You can camp on either side of the high-tide beach cutoff.

One of the best campsites on this beach sits on the top of the bluff, directly above the high-tide cutoff at Km. 27.8. To reach it, start at the west side of the high-tide cutoff, walk up the tree-trunk stairs, and follow the little trail to the top of the bluff. The campsite on this bluff offers you a commanding view of the entire beach. Logs and shrubs shelter the site from wind. If campers already occupy this spot, you can find several other choice campsites to the east and west of the high-tide cutoff.

During previous years, squatters occupied Central Sombrio Beach, but in the late 1990s, most of the beach returned to its natural state with the formation of the Juan de Fuca Marine Trail.

The beautiful sandy point directly west of the high-tide cutoff sits directly in front of the surfing area. The shoreline forms the kind of large, breaking waves that surfers and kayakers seek.

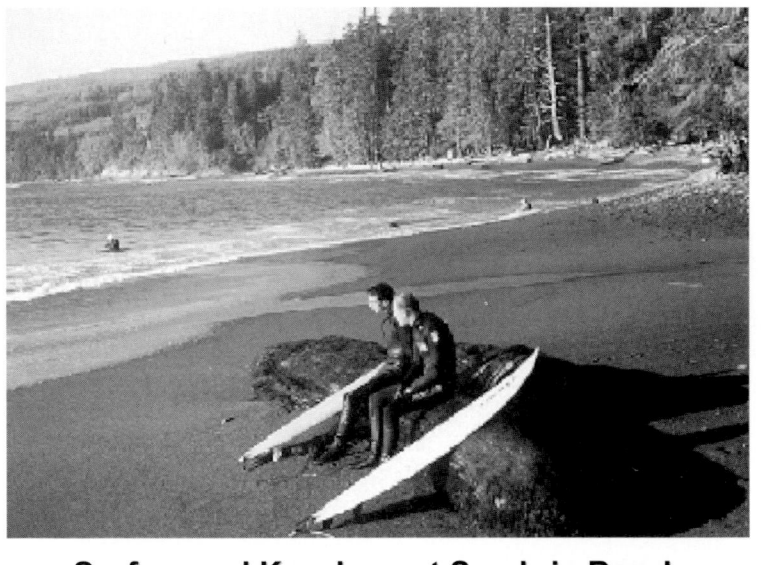

Surfers and Kayakers at Sombrio Beach

Continue hiking toward Sombrio River on the beach, or use the Trail in the forest. A Trail route cuts through the forest just west of the surfer's area. The **forest trail** leads to the suspension bridge and the parking lot. The **beach route** takes you to Sombrio River, where a path leads you to the suspension bridge. Before the installation of the suspension bridge, hikers had to ford the cold waters at the mouth of Sombrio River. *Note: If for any reason you need to exit the Trail at Sombrio Beach, go to the suspension bridge and up to the Sombrio Beach trailhead parking lot.*

From the suspension bridge, take the time to explore around the central beach area, and stretch your back. *Keep your socks clean and dry. Remember to bring the proper first aid in your pack in case of a blister.*

On the west side of the Sombrio River suspension bridge, continue down to the beach on a pleasant little trail. A campsite perched on the point beside the mouth of the river makes a perfect spot to pitch a tent.

The next section of the Trail abounds with interesting exploration possibilities. Those hikers wishing to complete the entire Trail in four days will want to continue on to Little Kuitsche Creek Campground. If you just hiked from Chin Beach, you may see the wisdom of staying at Sombrio Beach for the night. At Sombrio, you can explore, watch the sunset, enjoy a beach fire, and listen to the surf as you drift off to sleep. Open fires remain a beach privilege. Light your beach fires only below the high-tide mark. Campfire bans, occurring during dry spells in the summer months, apply to open fires everywhere.

D. SOMBRIO BEACH TO PARKINSON CREEK

Distance:	8 kilometres (Km. 29 to Km. 37)
Difficulty Rating:	intermediate
Average Hiking Time:	from 4 to 6 hours
Description of Trail:	boulder beach; rough, dense, low-bush trail; forest; old logging road; trail above cliff; views; boardwalk
Camping:	beach camping Km. 27.5; forest camping at Km. 33
High-tide Beach Cutoff:	at Km. 29.6 and Km. 30.2

This section covers the Trail from Sombrio Beach to Parkinson Creek. You may want to consider your camping options due to the lack of camping at Parkinson Creek. Between Sombrio Beach and Botanical Beach, designated campsites exist only at Little Kuitsche Creek and Payzant Creek. Whale watching from the cliff will entice you to camp at Little Kuitsche Creek (Km. 33). On the other hand, Payzant Creek (Km. 40) offers cascading waterfalls. In either case, be sure to leave plenty of time to explore the Parkinson Creek area.

When you reach the beach from the Trail heading west from the Sombrio River suspension bridge, you'll find that an information board displays only a tide guide, along with bear and cougar information. *Remember to wear bells or make noise to avoid surprising the larger species of wildlife.*

Huge boulders completely cover **West Sombrio Beach (Km. 29)**. The boulders present a challenge to trekkers with full packs. *A walking stick for balance makes hiking easier. Telescopic ski poles or cane-type umbrellas prove very useful for this trail. Bring one of these with you, because you will probably use it often.*

At Km. 29.6 on Sombrio Beach, a cliff towers above the beach. When the tide rises high, big waves flood the **high-tide cutoff** at the cliff. Fortunately, an alternate route circumnavigates the cliff cutoff area. Morning dew or rain can render the **alternate forest route** very slippery, so take special care if you use the forest detour around the cliff. A marker ball on either side of the cliff marks where you can access the alternate forest route.

At low tide, continue on the **beach route**. Keep your balance walking over the slippery beach rocks located directly below the cliff. Continue hiking on the boulder beach for another half kilometre. When you come to the next marker ball in a tree, you will also see the information board where the Trail continues into the forest.

The next three kilometres of Trail, characterized by six-metre-high trees, thick underbrush, and stumps, twist and turn through the new-growth forest all the way to Little Kuitsche Creek. When thick fog blankets the forest, the water droplets make conditions wet and slippery. The Trail hugs the ocean close enough for you to hear it, but you seldom enjoy a good view of the Juan de Fuca Strait. Draw your water for drinking from pools in a creek at Km. 30.1.

As you near the suspension bridge at **Minute Creek (Km. 32)**, listen for the sound of the waterfall resounding through the forest. To the east of the creek (about 122 metres), before the gorge, find the little path to the shoreline and to the mouth of the creek. Expect a long climb down to the creekbed below. It is well worth the trouble. *Wear your reef boots if you plan to visit the waterfall.* Take a rest at Minute Creek, enjoy the view, and explore the area. If you plan to camp for the night at Little Kuitsche Creek, you can decide how much time remains for exploring before hiking to the campground a kilometre away.

A half-kilometre west of Minute Creek (Km. 32.5) you will see a rocky clearing where you can sit, rest, and enjoy one of nature's little wonders. I call this spot Thunder Rock Blowhole. Waves rushing into a tunnel-like surge channel make a rumble like thunder and force the saltwater spray out the other end. I stop to enjoy this spot every time I hike here. If you want to stay dry, do not get close. When you least expect it, a big wave will come thundering in, and the ocean spray will explode out of the rocky blowhole.

Continue to where the boardwalks at **Little Kuitsche Creek (Km. 33)** welcome you to the campground. The information board displays a map of the camp area. Just north of the information board, you will find the pit toilets and a little trail that leads to a stream where you can draw fresh water for drinking and cooking.

Campsite pads are in the tall bushes around a circular trail. As you walk around the camp area, choose a camping spot that you like. *Use a camp stove for hot food preparation at forest campsites. Open fires in the forest carry hefty fines and may cause a forest fire. Be smart and use your camp stove when cooking in the forest.* Beside the campground, a lookout area perched on a rock at the shoreline treats hikers to a peaceful place to watch a sunset or look for whales. Hikers staying overnight might wish to take a short evening walk to Kuitsche Creek, a ten-minute walk west of Little Kuitsche Creek. *Carry a flashlight on evening walks.*

Kuitsche Creek has a beach that welcomes exploration. Be careful as you make your way down to the waterfalls and pools below the bridge. Instead of climbing down the dangerously slippery rocks of the streambed, use the path in front of the bridge, which climbs up, around, and down to the hidden beach via a trail. Beach camping can be fun on this secluded, seldom-used beach. *To avoid getting swamped by a rising tide in the middle of the night, camp well above the highest high-tide mark.*

West of Km. 34, a thin strip of old-growth trees stands along the bluff beside the Trail. Ladders, bridges, big cedar trees, and views of the Juan de Fuca Strait await you as the Trail leads away from the ocean and up into the clearing around deep gorges that follow the shoreline. Hiking along the bluff gives you an opportunity to enjoy the views of the Juan de Fuca Strait. A few rest areas allow you to relax and watch for whales and other marine life.

The Trail becomes less erratic after Km. 36, and boardwalks lead you up to the road near **Parkinson Creek (Km. 37)**. Travel west along the road past Km. 37 and on to the double-post gate near the Parkinson Creek trailhead parking lot, trail information signs, and pit toilets. Currently, Parkinson Creek lacks a designated campground. <u>Camp there only in a **real emergency** situation or you could be **fined**.</u> Take note of the little overgrown road where the Trail road curves up to the parking lot. That little road leads to the beginning of the path to the seal grotto. Walk for 35 paces down the overgrown road to make a note of where the seal grotto path begins. At the end of the overgrown road, find a spot to set up a tent. Draw fresh water from Parkinson Creek, a five-minute walk along the main hiking road west of the parking lot.

To locate another suitable camping spot, go west from the parking lot on the road to Parkinson Creek bridge. Follow the Trail signs left down the gravel trail that follows parallel to Parkinson Creek. To find the camping spot that trekkers only should use in a real emergency, take this gravel trail to its end. Before the end of the gravel trail, you will see a sign indicating the continuation of the Juan de Fuca Marine Trail.

Be sure to allow time on your hike to explore the Parkinson Creek area before continuing to Payzant Creek campsite or Botanical Beach. *See Chapter 6: Hidden Treasures, #9 - Seal Grotto, Tide Pools, and Falls (at Km. 38) for more information about the Parkinson Creek seal grotto.*

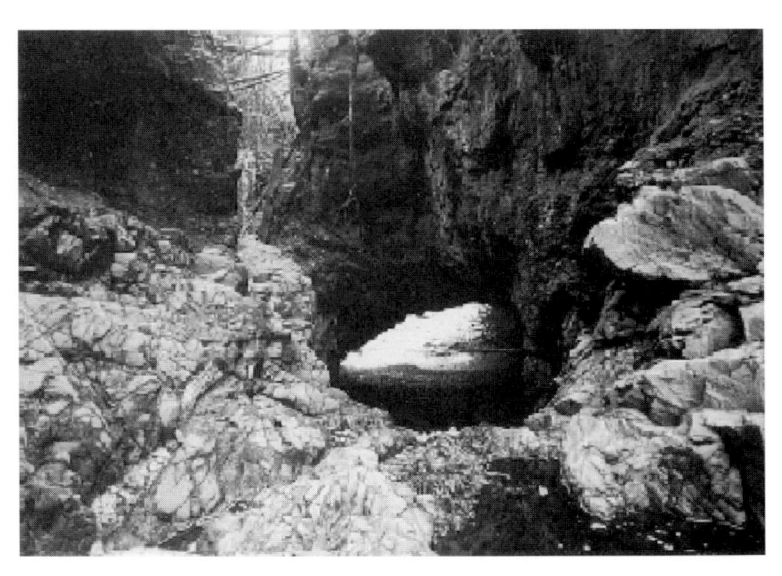

Seal Grotto at Parkinson Creek

E. PARKINSON CREEK TO BOTANICAL BEACH TRAILHEAD

Distance:	10 kilometres (Km. 37 to Km. 47)
Difficulty Rating:	intermediate
Average Hiking Time:	from 4 to 6 hours
Description of Trail:	logging road, mature forest, reef shelf, beach
Forest Camping:	at Payzant Creek
High-tide Beach Cutoff:	Tide pools are visible at tides below 1.2 metres. There are no high-tide cutoffs west of Km. 31.0.

The most interesting section of the Juan de Fuca Marine Trail lies directly ahead. The rocky reef between Km. 38 and Km. 39 beckons us to be a little adventurous and explore with abandon. Payzant Creek's waterfall entices all to take a long look and welcomes us to stay overnight at the campsite. The beautiful, peaceful seclusion of Providence Cove is hard to leave. Along the way, you will pass by inaccessible hidden beaches, rock arches, and rugged reefs. Beautiful tide pools at Botanical Beach make us want to drop those heavy packs and explore on the reef.

If you arrived at **Parkinson Creek trailhead** from either Sombrio Beach or Little Kuitsche Creek, you may want to consider camping at Payzant Creek for the night. The three-kilometre hike from Parkinson Creek to Payzant Creek campsite takes about an hour to hike. Those trekkers who started their trek from Botanical Beach should also consider staying at Payzant Creek if they wish to spend extra time the next day exploring the reef shelf and the Parkinson Creek area.

From Parkinson Creek parking lot, follow the old logging road west past two bridges, the second one being the **Parkinson Creek bridge**. Next, follow the signs guiding you left, down the path, which parallels Parkinson Creek. After a short hike, you arrive at the Trail sign indicating the continuation of the Juan de Fuca Marine Trail.

The next half-kilometre of Trail passes through an area of short trees, shrubs, and underbrush. A few large trees become visible along the shoreline. At Km. 38, the Trail puts you onto the reef shelf by the ocean. *Wear bells in this area to avoid a run-in with a bear or cougar.*

After Km. 38, when on the reef, you get a very close view of the ocean and surf rolling your way. Tide pools dot this reef shelf, so take

41

advantage of the viewing opportunity if you arrive here at low tide. Whales, seals, and other mammals often swim by. You will spot a beach marker ball eighty metres to the west of your entrance onto the reef. Here you can decide either to walk on the **reef shelf** or to get back onto the **forest trail**. If the tide rises high, do not take the reef, because it will surely block your passage at a low shelf a half-kilometre west of Km. 38. If the rising tide does block your way, simply go back to the previous marker ball near Km. 38 and take the forest trail.

If you continue hiking on the **reef shelf**, do so only at low tide, and keep a sharp lookout for rogue waves. Continue on to the first marker ball at Km. 39, and then return to the forest trail. You will see only one marker ball on the reef at Km. 39. No marker balls hang beyond this point. If you stay on the reef shelf past this last marker ball, more impassable spots farther on will block your route and force you to return. Hiking can be tricky on the reef shelf, but it is definitely a lot of fun. After exploring the reef, you must return to the forest trail at Km. 39.

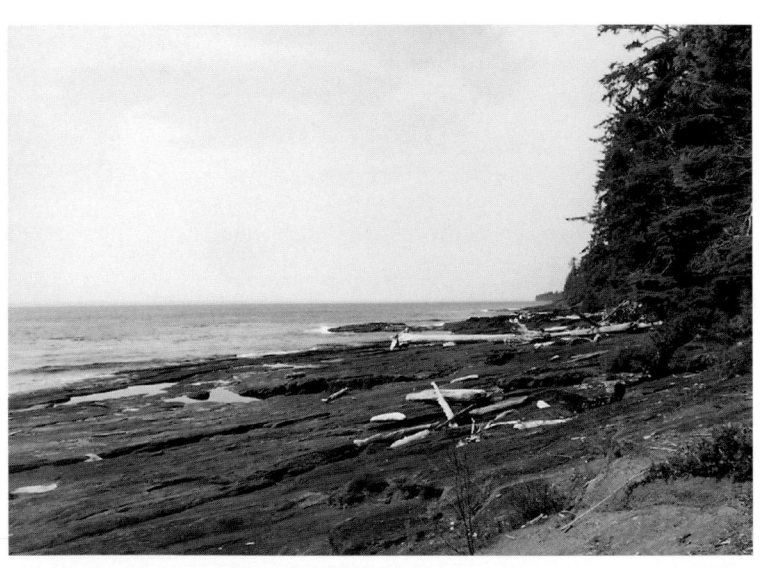

Reef Shelf at Km. 38

If the tide is high, you will have to continue hiking on the **forest trail**. You will soon leave the new growth area and enter the medium-growth forest, where boardwalks make the walking easy.

Payzant Creek Campground (Km. 40) greets you with a spectacular view of a waterfall cascading into a large pool near the Trail. The information board shows the layout of the camping area. *Choose a camping pad with good drainage, just in case it rains during the night.*

Providence Cove, located one kilometre west of Payzant Creek, hides between two towering cliffs. The Trail, at the approach to Providence Cove, follows a bluff near the cove and then crosses over **Yauh Creek**. Stairs carved into a tree follow down its trunk and across the creek. Pools of crystal-clear water make Yauh Creek a good spot from which to draw water. Obey the signs that warn you not to camp or light fires at or near Providence Cove. Take the time to visit its picturesque cliff-protected beach. For many centuries, native people used this spot as a hunting camp.

Continue hiking past Providence Cove where the Trail becomes level and enjoyable. A few roots and logs may hinder your progress in this forest of medium-growth trees. *Avoid stepping on slippery roots and wet logs. Step over them and avoid a fall.*

Just when you least expect it, the Trail, at Km. 41.5, leads you to a little, exposed shelf on the rocky shore. This time, the going gets rough. Follow along the steep rocky bluff about a hundred metres to the next marker ball. From this perch, on a clear day you can see the Pacific Ocean. Do not continue hiking on the reef shelf. The rough shoreline walk on the reef becomes slow going for those carrying a heavy pack. Continue hiking on the forest trail because the Trail hugs the shoreline close enough for you to enjoy the views. Km. 41.6 leads out to a point overlooking the ocean and would make a fine spot for a rest. A little farther on, at low tide, you may spot another rock arch down at the shoreline. At high tide, the arch becomes submerged.

At Km. 42.5, the Trail crosses a stream and then immediately turns back up into the forest. At that point, a beach marker ball hangs in a tree over the small, ten-metre section of beach trail. If you go exploring on the reef shelf, look for these marker balls in order to find your way back to the forest trail.

Further along, **Soule Creek (Km. 43.1)** greets you with a sturdy wooden bridge, freshwater pools, and many little waterfalls. The Trail follows the streambed toward the ocean bluffs, where boardwalks make walking easy.

When walking up on the bluffs (Km. 44), you get a commanding view of the ocean. Only two more kilometres of reef and beach lie ahead of you before the Trail turns upward from Km. 46 to the wide gravel path leading to the Botanical Beach parking lot and the end of your trek.

Start enjoying the tide pools, and get onto the reef at your first opportunity, near **Tom Baird Creek (Km. 44.5)**. To see the tide pools, be sure you time your hike to arrive at low tide.

If the tide is high, stay on the **forest trail.** When high tide comes in, the ocean floods the reef and beach, making exploring the tide pools impossible. If the tide is low, you can trek on the **reef shelf** to a little island. Detour behind the island to avoid getting too close to the surge channel situated on the west side of the island.

Botanical Beach begins at Km. 45. The tide pool area begins just past Km. 46 and continues all the way to Botany Bay. If you want to see the marine life in the tide pools, you must plan ahead to arrive at Botanical Beach at extreme low tides. To see the tide pools at low tide, you must get right out onto the reef shelf when the tide is below 1.2 metres. In the tide pools, you might see such marine animals as sea urchins, sea cucumbers, shore crabs, hermit crabs, octopus, starfish, mussels, chitons, limpets, sea anemones, sculpins, barnacles, and periwinkles. Marine plants include algae, rockweed, surf grass, and sea sacs.

Picnic tables at Km. 46 provide a great place to rest and eat. You can examine the interesting tide pool photograph, which identifies many of the species of marine life living in the tide pools.

If time and energy permit, follow the special trail around Botanical Beach called the Shoreline Trail to the tide pool Special Feature Zone. This zone is located on the exposed reef and has thousands of tide pools of all sizes to enjoy. *For more information about the tide pools, the Shoreline Trail and Botany Bay, see Chapter 6: Hidden Treasures, #9 - Tides Pools (at Km. 46).*

Hikers wanting to go directly to the parking lot should follow the signs from Km. 46 up the wide, one-kilometre-long gravel path. At last, you arrive at the **Botanical Beach (Km. 47)** parking lot. The entire Botanical Beach area, including the parking lot, is restricted to day use only.

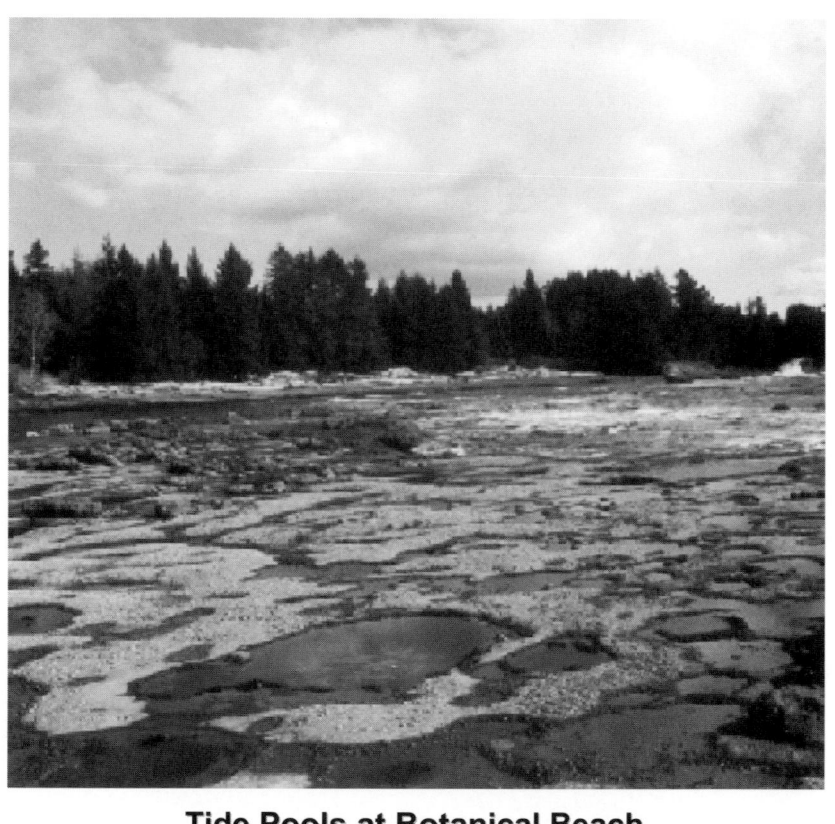

Tide Pools at Botanical Beach

After the trek, weary hikers usually go to the hotels, restaurants, and camping areas in nearby Port Renfrew, which is four kilometres from the Botanical Beach parking lot. The friendly people of Port Renfrew are well versed in receiving hikers from the Juan de Fuca Marine Trail who want to eat, relax, and dream about their hike. Hikers may even dream about returning again next year.

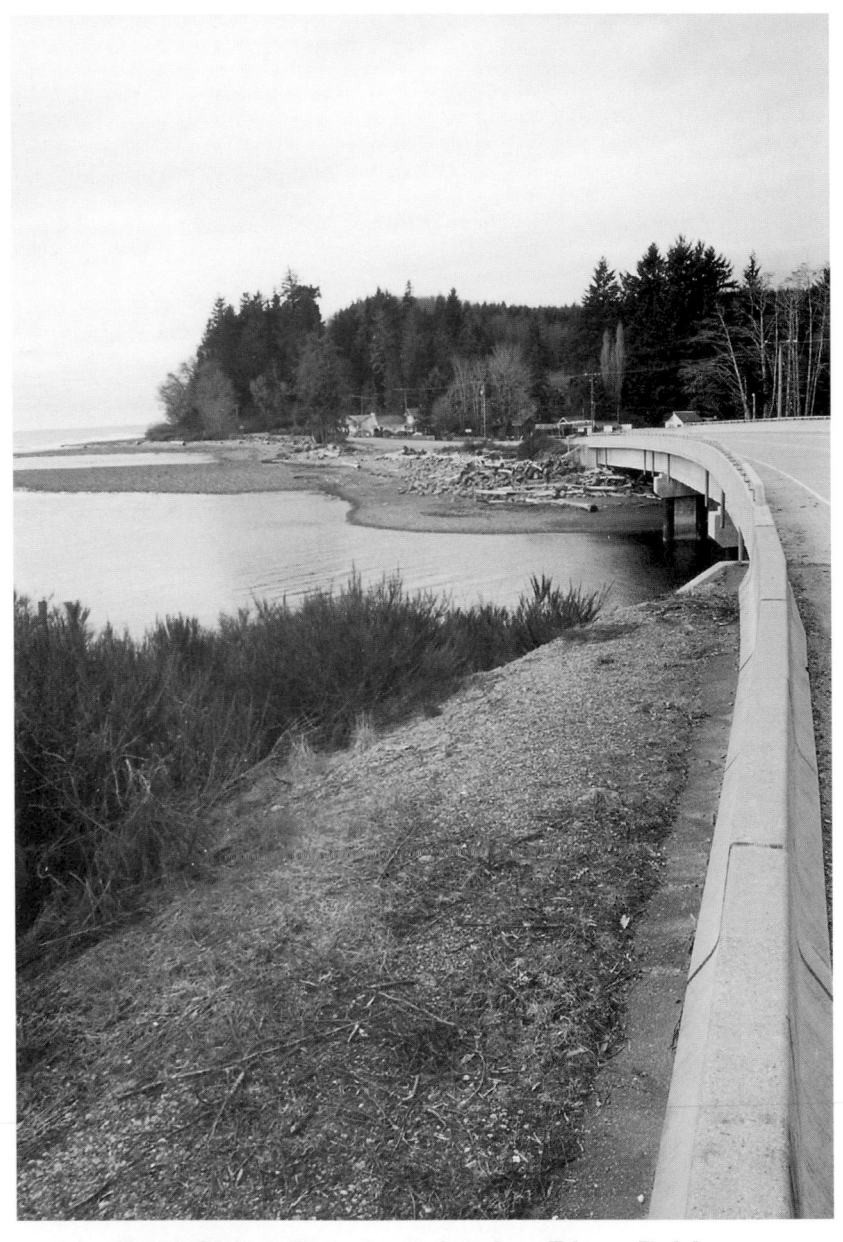

East China Beach at Jordan River Bridge

Chapter 4
Options to Extend Your Trek

The Juan de Fuca Marine Trail usually takes four or five days to trek completely. This chapter will serve those trekkers who want to extend the enjoyment of their hike by adding one or all of the following options described in this chapter. Hiking teams wanting to embark upon a grand, two-trail super trek of 122 kilometres can combine the West Coast Trail with the Juan de Fuca Marine Trail.

1. JORDAN RIVER PUBLIC CAMPGROUND TO CHINA BEACH TRAILHEAD

Distance:	adds 4 kilometres to the east end of your trek
Difficulty Rating:	easy to intermediate
Average Hiking Time:	from 1.5 hours to 2 hours
Description of Trail:	beach hike, then ½ kilometre on forest trail
Beach Camping:	no beach camping; day use only
High-tide Beach Cutoff:	China Beach may be under water when the tide rises above 3 metres. Check the tide guide before your hike.

You can add four extra kilometres on beautiful China Beach to the east end of your trek of the Juan de Fuca Marine Trail. Start your trek at the Jordan River campground, located in the town of Jordan River beside the Jordan River bridge. Enjoy the views from this prime oceanfront property, located along Highway #14 in the center of the town. This public area offers free camping and free parking on a first-come, first-serve basis.

You may park your vehicle in the parking area for the duration of your trek. Begin your trek by crossing the Jordan River bridge and walk west on Highway #14 for about a hundred metres, where you take the short path leading onto the beach. When you reach it, trek for 3.5 kilometres west along the beach. On arriving near the west end of China Beach, you will see pit toilets that mark where the trail leads up into the forest and to the lower China Beach parking lot.

A fifteen-minute, half-kilometre hike through the old-growth forest brings you to the lower China Beach parking lot. Walk west for four minutes to the upper parking lot, the official Juan de Fuca Marine Trail trailhead. Before continuing your trek read the bulletin board, then deposit your camping fee in the deposit box located at the trailhead (Km. 0) in the parking lot. Please read the rules regarding camping and fees on the information board. From this point, you continue west on the main Juan de Fuca Marine Trail.

2.   BOTANY BAY/BOTANICAL BEACH TRAIL LOOP

Distance:	adds 1 extra kilometre to the west end of your trek
Difficulty Rating:	easy to intermediate
Average Hiking Time:	from 1 to 2 hours
Description of Trail:	beach hike, tide pool reef shelf, and a forest hike on gentle terrain
Camping:	no beach or forest camping at Botanical Beach, day use only; camp in Port Renfrew at designated campgrounds
Tide Pool Observation:	best when tides below 1.2 metres

Add one kilometre to your hike by using this trail loop. Instead of hiking from Km. 46 directly to the Botanical Beach parking lot at Km. 47, take the stairs down to the Shoreline Trail Loop. The loop passes Botany Bay and then continues up to the parking lot (Km. 47). You will find picnic tables at Botanical Beach at Km. 46 and at the parking lot. If you want to view the renowned Botanical Beach tide pools, time your hike to arrive at Botanical Beach at low tide. Tide pool observation is best when the tides are below 1.2 metres. You will find pit toilets located along the trail near Botany Bay and at the parking lot.

To view the tide pools, walk out onto the large reef shelf west of Km. 46, and continue walking west beside the tide pools for a kilometre until you nearly reach Botany Bay. Be cautious and avoid falling into the tide pools. The reef rocks are very slippery. Watch for the rising tide and rogue waves. When on the tide pool reef, if you look up at the trees you will see the red marker balls, which indicate the locations where you can return to the Shoreline Trail.

See the map of the Botanical Beach, Botany Bay and Mill Bay area in Chapter 6: Hidden Treasures, #9 - Tide Pools (at Km. 46).

3. WEST COAST TRAIL

Distance:	adds 75 kilometres
Difficulty Rating:	difficult, for experts only
Average Hiking Time:	from 6 to 9 days
Description of Trail:	See "West Coast Trail Hiker Preparation Guide" at www.sookenet.com/sooke/activity/trails
Reservations, Fees:	1-800-663-6000 (Canada, USA); 1-250-387-1643 (elsewhere)

The West Coast Trail, a part of the Pacific Rim National Park Reserve, belongs to Canada's National Park System. This trail, recommended for expert hikers only, opens May 1 and closes September 30 of each year. Phone one of the above numbers for complete details on fees. The West Coast Trail Hiker Preparation Guide is now required reading before hiking the trail. You can view it at the Internet site mentioned above. If you have no access to the Internet, the reservation office will mail the guide to you, along with a trail map, when you make reservations to hike the trail.

With good planning, you can combine the Juan de Fuca Marine Trail with the West Coast Trail. Start with either trek, and when you finish the first leg, recharge your pack with more food for the second leg. To replenish your food supplies, a good plan would include arrangements to pick up your food cache in Port Renfrew. Plan and practice all aspects of the trip before attempting the grand two-trail super trek.

Commence your West Coast Trail hike at either Port Renfrew or Bamfield. Phone the Juan de Fuca Express in Port Renfrew (see Appendix) for jet boat transportation service to and from Bamfield and Port Renfrew. Be sure to reserve your spot to hike the West Coast Trail before you commence the two-trail super trek.

Take advantage of the daily bus service available to hikers. Contact the West Coast Trail Express Bus by phone or e-mail (see Appendix). When hiking, be sure to let someone know your itinerary.

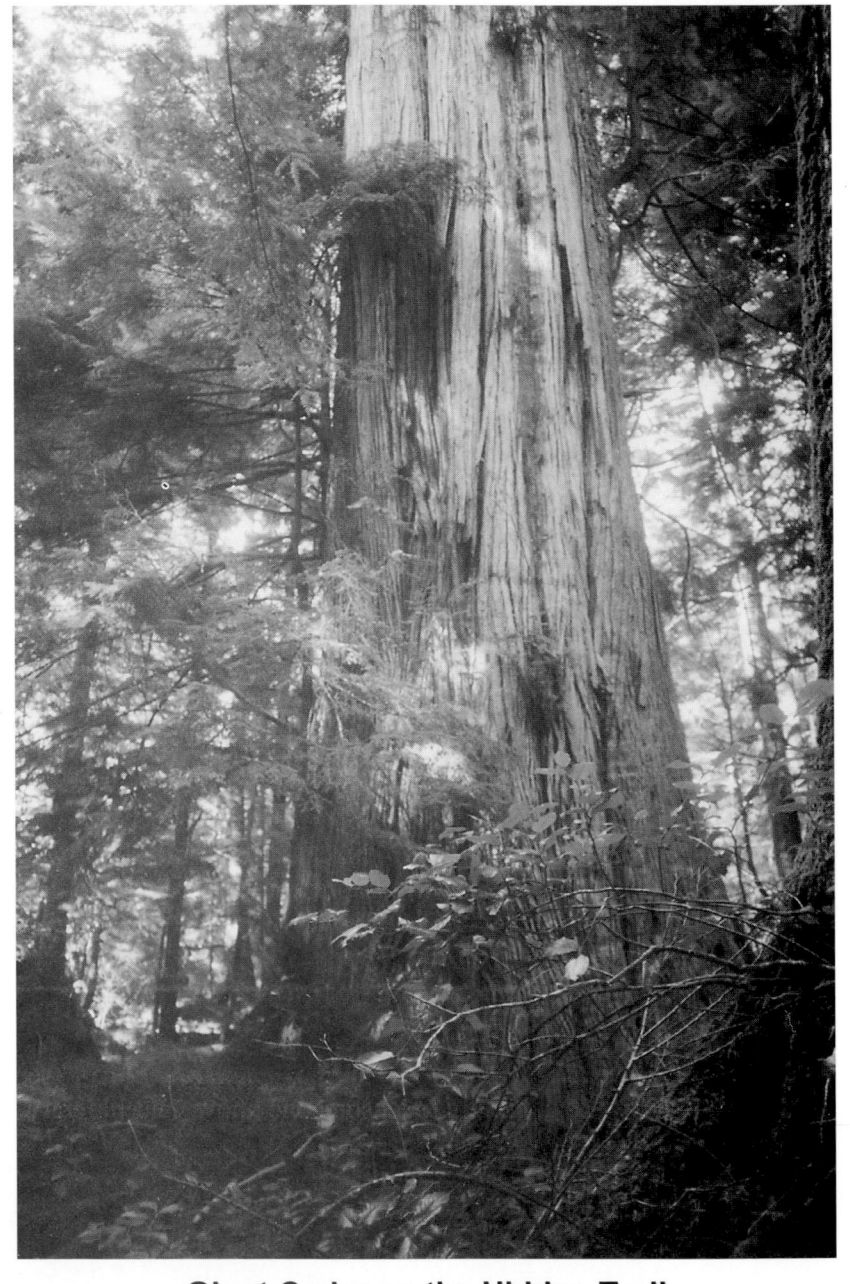

Giant Cedar on the Hidden Trail

Chapter 5
Unmarked Side Trails

Some rough trails and old overgrown logging roads lead from Highway #14 to the main Juan de Fuca Marine Trail. Although they **do not** belong to the Juan de Fuca Marine Trail system, they can provide emergency access to and from the Trail.

Hikers unaware of the unmarked side trails can make only short return-type walks from either of the trailheads, but those who know about these side trails can effectively day hike the Juan de Fuca Marine Trail. One-way day hikes and one-way weekend or overnight hikes between China Beach and Sombrio Beach would be impossible without using at least one of the side trails as an entry or exit point. These side trails could make the Juan de Fuca Marine Trail completely accessible and many times more useful to day hikers and weekend or overnight hikers.

As with all trails in any forest, these unmarked trails become very slippery and potentially dangerous when wet from rain, fog, mist, and morning dew. Some of these side trails include steep sections.

It will be useful to know the location of the side trails if you have an emergency along the trail. You could draw these five side trails on your colour map of the Juan De Fuca Marine Trail. This would also give you a better idea of how long it will take you to complete your day hikes and overnight or weekend hikes, if you decide to use these side trails as entry or exit points. **Be aware that the gated logging roads and some of the unmarked side trails are on private property. Use them at your own liability, and at your own risk.**

The following pages contain maps and descriptions of these five unmarked side trails.

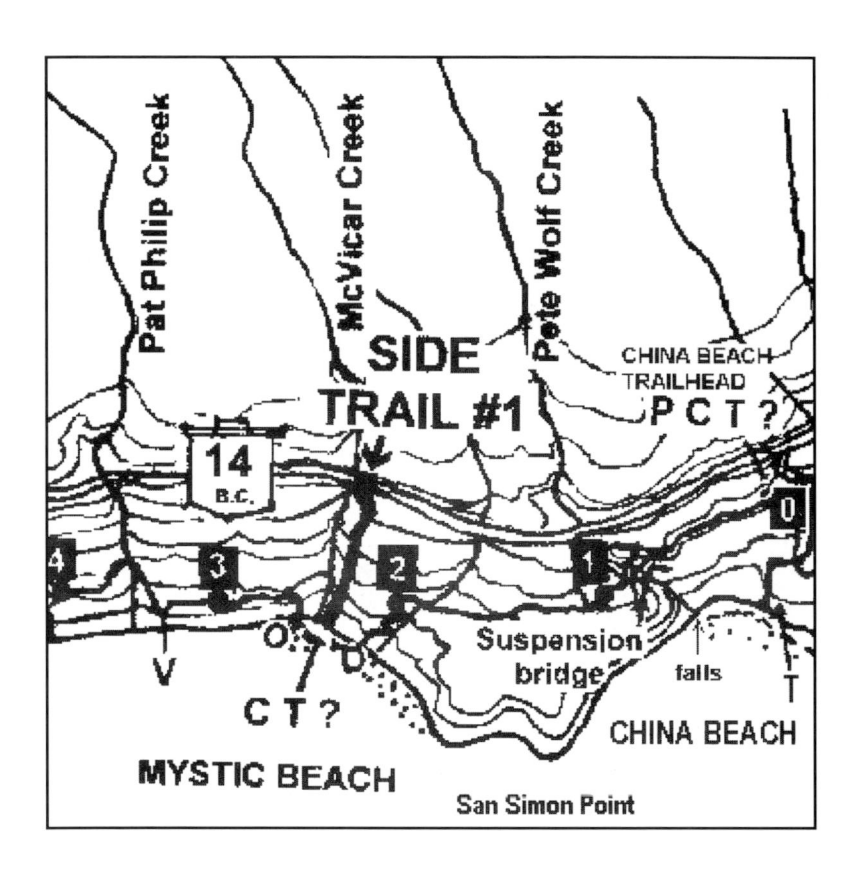

Unmarked Side Trail #1

Mystic Beach at Km. 2.6

UNMARKED SIDE TRAIL #1: MYSTIC BEACH AT KM. 2.6

The main Juan de Fuca Marine Trail from China Beach trailhead to Mystic Beach is 2.5 kilometres and takes approximately forty-five minutes to hike. You could hike the half kilometre from Highway #14 to Mystic Beach within fifteen minutes using the side trail.

Location:

The side trail connects Mystic Beach at Trail Km. 2.6 with Highway #14 at McVicar Creek bridge on Highway #14.

Finding the side trail from the Juan de Fuca Marine Trail:

You may encounter difficulty locating the unmarked side trail when hiking on Mystic Beach. Start by going to the west end of Mystic Beach, and locate the trail information sign and beach access marker ball at Km. 2.6. Take note of the two large truck-sized boulders on the beach in front of the information signs at McVicar Creek. From the boulders and trail signs, walk 60 paces along the beach in an easterly direction. You should be able to locate a little unmarked side trail that leads into the low bushes. The side trail veers to the left for several metres and then climbs up into the forest. Use caution at the broken stairs on the lower end of the trail. A hundred metres farther up, on the flatter part of the forest floor, the side trail leads up to Highway #14.

Getting to the side trail from Highway #14:

Drive west 1.8 kilometres from the turnoff at China Beach trailhead along Highway #14 to the McVicar Creek bridge. The side trail meets Highway #14 approximately fifteen metres east of the McVicar Creek bridge. Use extra caution at the steep section near the beach. Remember exactly where the side trail comes out on the beach, in case you need to return the same way, back to Highway #14.

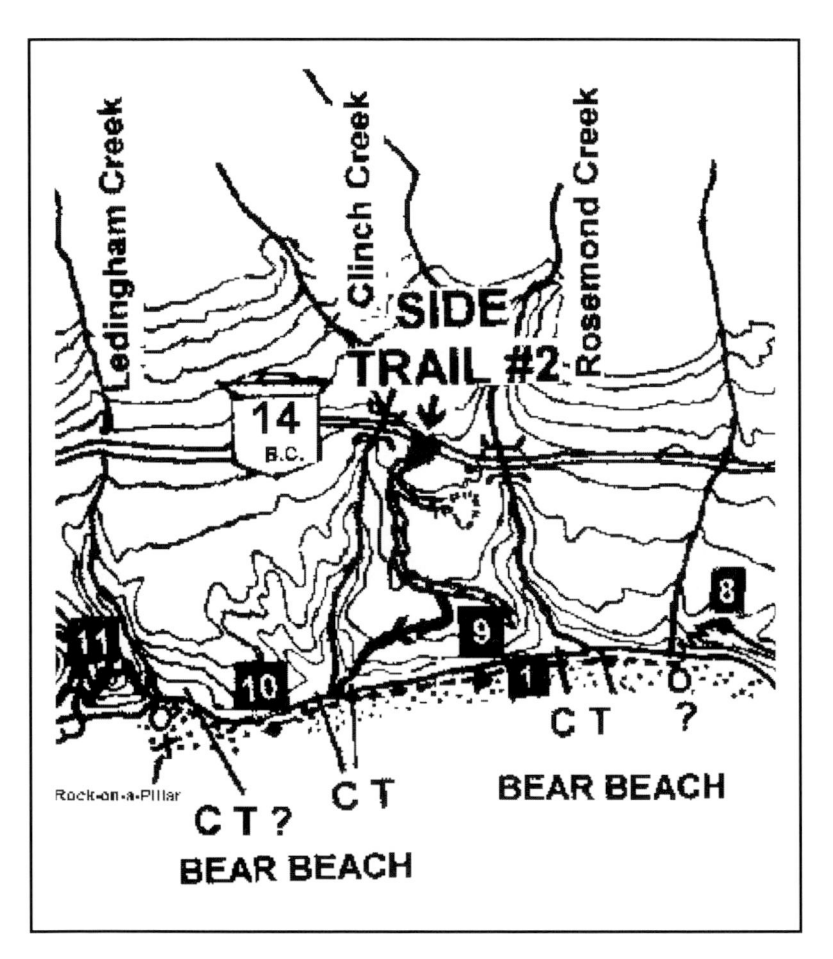

Unmarked Side Trail #2

Clinch Creek at Km. 9.6

UNMARKED SIDE TRAIL #2: CLINCH CREEK AT KM. 9.6

Bear Beach is in the middle of an isolated stretch on the Juan de Fuca Marine Trail. Hiking to Bear Beach takes five hours from China Beach trailhead and two days from Sombrio Beach. You could hike from Highway #14 to Bear Beach in ten minutes using the side trail.

Location:

The side trail connects Clinch Creek on Bear Beach at Km. 9.6 with Highway #14 at the gated road just east of Clinch Creek bridge on Highway #14.

Finding the side trail from the Juan de Fuca Marine Trail:

The unmarked side trail near Clinch Creek is at Km. 9.6 on Bear Beach, 35 paces east of the mouth of Clinch Creek. Find the trail that leads into the woods over roots, logs, and boards. Take the right fork. A dozen metres along the trail, you must climb up a steep, four-metre embankment. The trail continues to climb steeply up a ridge for forty metres and then levels out. Eventually, the trail joins an old logging road. You will see a tree painted with white and black squares. Follow the road to the west (left), where it joins another gravel road about two hundred metres farther on. At the intersection of the two roads, you will see a boulder painted with one black and one white square. Follow the second road left, and you will come to the yellow gate at Highway #14, just past the gravel pits.

Getting to the side trail from Highway #14:

Locate the old gated gravel pit road between Clinch Creek and Rosemond Creek, about 6.6 kilometres along Highway #14 from the turnoff at China Beach trailhead. On the other side of the highway, look for a twenty-centimeter sign with a numeral 3 on it. Do not park in front of the yellow gate. Instead, park on the north side of Highway #14. Follow the road past the quarry. Halfway around the first corner, a second road leads off to the right. Take the second road south. There you will pass a rock with black-and-white markings. Ten minutes down the second road on the right-hand (south) side, on the long level section in the woods, you will see a path beside a tree with black-and-white paint. The path leads down to Clinch Creek on Bear Beach.

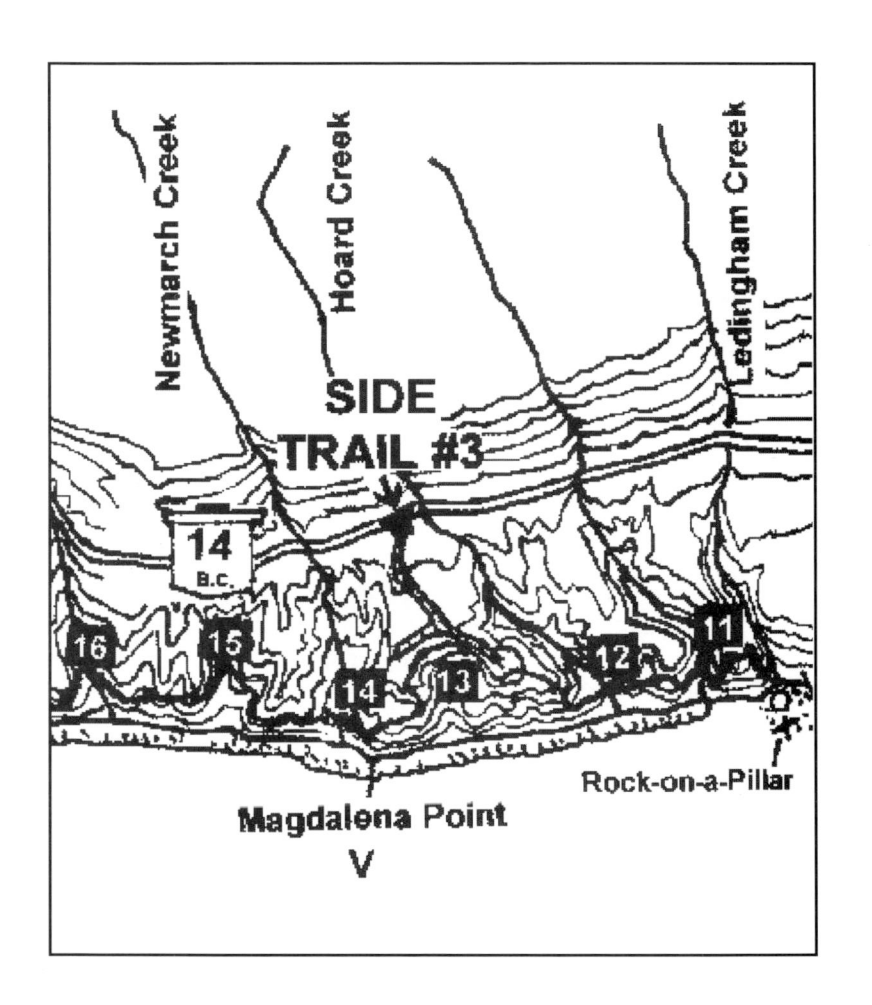

Unmarked Side Trail #3

Magdalena Point at Km. 13

UNMARKED SIDE TRAIL #3: MAGDALENA POINT AT KM. 13

Magdalena Point is in the middle of an isolated stretch on the Juan de Fuca Marine Trail. Hiking to Magdalena Point takes eight hours from China Beach trailhead and ten hours from Sombrio Beach. You could hike from Highway #14 to Magdalena Point in twenty minutes using the side trail. The mouth of Hoard Creek is only a thirty-minute walk away from Highway #14.

Location:

The side trail connects the Trail at Km. 13 with a logging road the leads to Highway #14.

Finding the side trail from the Juan de Fuca Marine Trail:

At Km. 13 near Magdalena Point, the Juan de Fuca Marine Trail is right beside an old logging road. It is only two metres from the Trail to the old logging road. To reach Highway #14, walk for only ten minutes from the south end of the road to the north end.

Getting to the side trail from Highway #14:

From the turnoff at the China Beach trailhead, drive 9.2 kilometres west along Highway #14, where you will see a gated road. On the other side of the highway, look for a twenty-centimeter sign with a numeral 4 on it. Locate the old gated road approximately two kilometres past Clinch Creek bridge. Do not park in front of the yellow gate. Follow the old gravel road for ten minutes down the left fork to the Juan de Fuca Marine Trail sign. Get onto the Trail at that point and you will see the marker for Km. 13 close by.

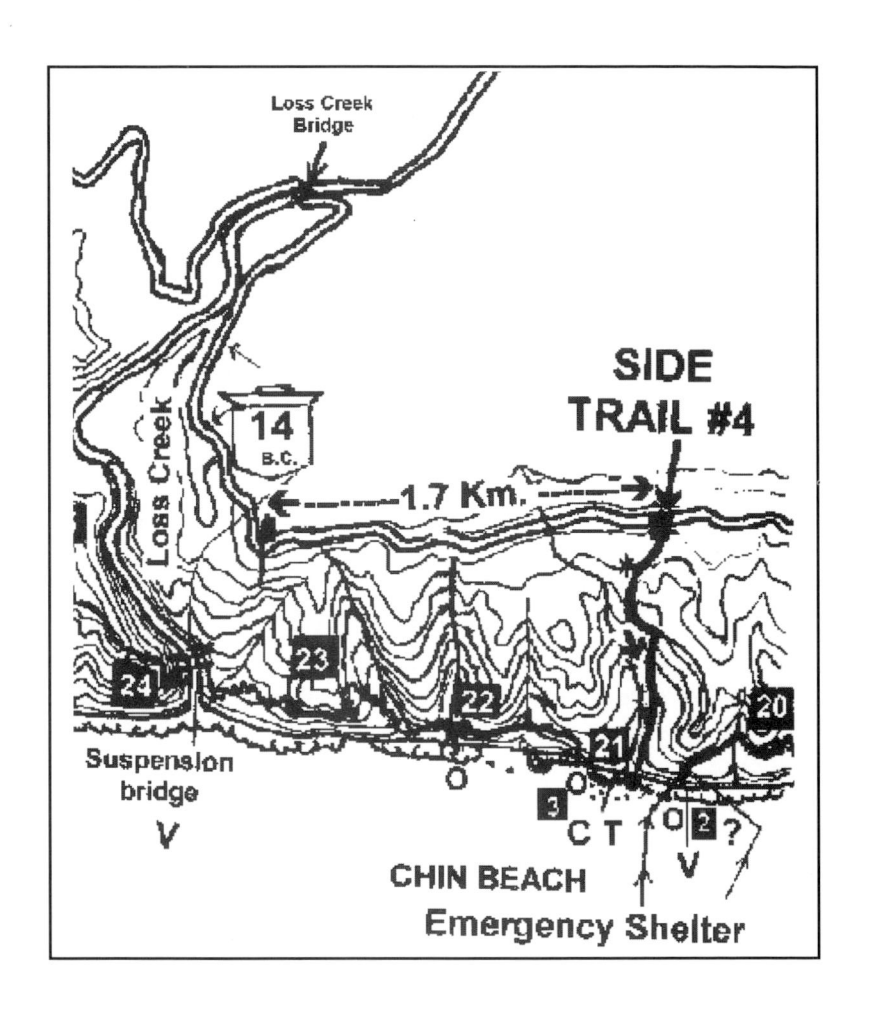

Unmarked Side Trail #4

Chin Beach at Km. 21

UNMARKED SIDE TRAIL #4: CHIN BEACH AT KM. 21

Chin Beach is in the middle of an isolated stretch on the Juan de Fuca Marine Trail. Hiking to Chin Beach takes two days from China Beach trailhead and four hours from Sombrio Beach. You could hike from Highway #14 to the giant cedar trees in ten minutes and to Chin Beach in forty minutes using the side trail.

Location:

The side trail connects Chin Beach at Km. 21 with Highway #14 via a hidden trail located approximately 1.7 kilometres east of the ninety-degree turn going down to the Loss Creek bridge along Highway #14.

Finding the side trail from the Juan de Fuca Marine Trail:

Find this unmarked side trail near Km. 21 on Chin Beach, just east of the toilets and stream. First, locate the campsite behind the Km. 21 marker, and follow the trail up into the forest. The first kilometre of the unmarked side trail leads uphill. Use caution here. After the steep climb, the trail levels out for the next kilometre and veers off to the left. Then it gradually tracks toward Highway #14. Hiking the two kilometres from Chin Beach to Highway #14 will take about forty minutes. Many old-growth giant cedars grow in this area of the forest.

Getting to the side trail from Highway #14:

Drive west from the turnoff at the China Beach trailhead for thirteen kilometres on Highway #14 and look for the two thirty-centimeter-long letters "H" and "T" painted on the highway in front of the entrance to the trail. The letters stand for Hidden Trail, and as you might expect, the trail may be difficult to locate (see map). Park your vehicle well off the highway. Follow the trail into the forest. After ten minutes of hiking, you will pass the giant cedar trees. Twenty minutes into the hike you will come to a steep slope that leads down to Km. 21. Hike for a total of forty to fifty minutes from Highway #14 down to Chin Beach. Remember that the side trail meets the beach directly behind the campsite behind the marker for Km. 21. Find the pit toilets thirty metres west of the marker.

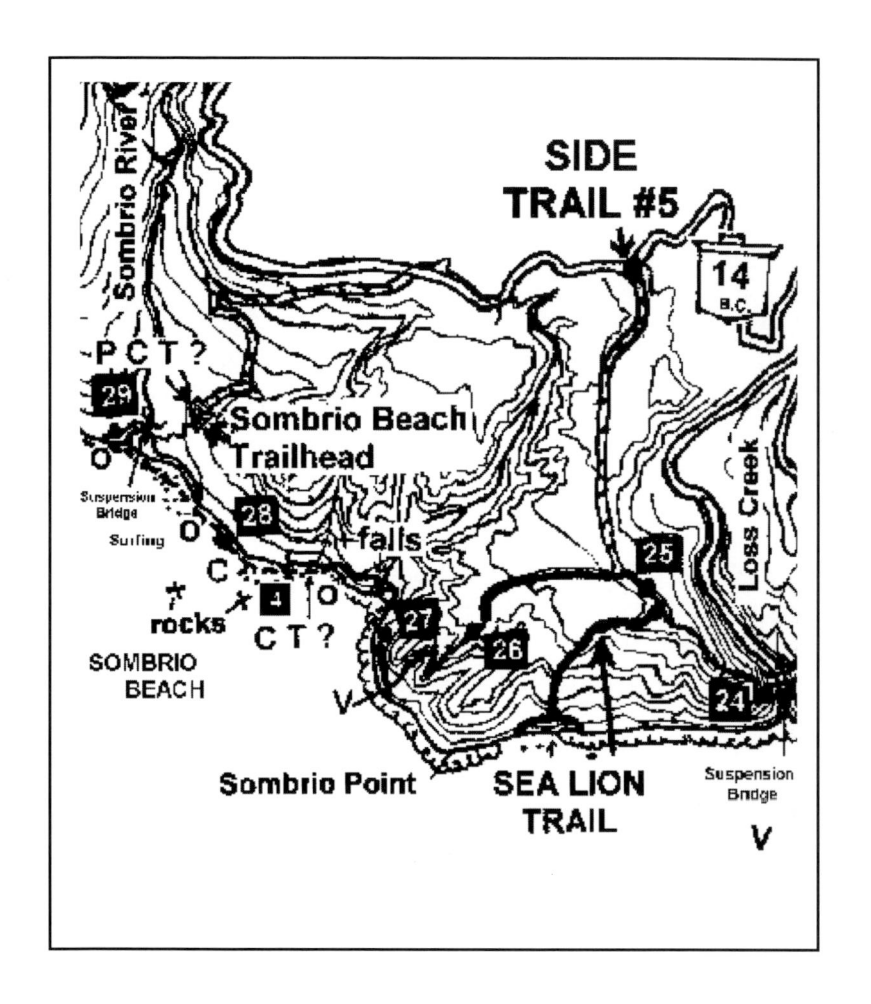

Unmarked Side Trail #5

Loss Creek at Km. 25

UNMARKED SIDE TRAIL #5: LOSS CREEK AT KM. 25

The Loss Creek suspension bridge and the sea lion caves, two very popular destinations, are located in the middle of an isolated stretch on the Juan de Fuca Marine Trail. Hiking to the Loss Creek suspension bridge takes two days from China Beach trailhead and two hours from Sombrio Beach. Using the side trail, you could hike to the Loss Creek area in thirty minutes.

Location:

The Juan de Fuca Marine Trail connects to an old logging road between Km. 25 and Km. 26. The old road also connects with Highway #14 two kilometres east of the Sombrio Road turnoff on Highway #14.

Finding the side trail from the Juan de Fuca Marine Trail:

When you reach the old logging road, find the trail marker for Km. 25. From there, walk to the fork in the road, and continue hiking for twenty minutes on the north fork up to Highway #14. You will pass an iron gate near Highway #14 that blocks the entrance to the old logging road.

Getting to the side trail from Highway #14:

Locate the old logging road and gate two kilometres west of the Loss Creek bridge on Highway #14. On the other side of Highway #14 from the gated road, look for a twenty-centimeter sign with a numeral 7 on it. Park your vehicle on the north side of the highway. Follow the old road for twenty minutes to the fork in the road. Take the left (east) fork to the trail marker at Km. 25. Near the end of this road, find the path leading down to the sea lion caves and islands.

Continue hiking to the end of the road (on the east fork) on the Juan de Fuca Marine Trail to get to the Loss Creek suspension bridge and gorge at Km. 24. The west fork of the road leads to Sombrio Point and Sombrio Beach.

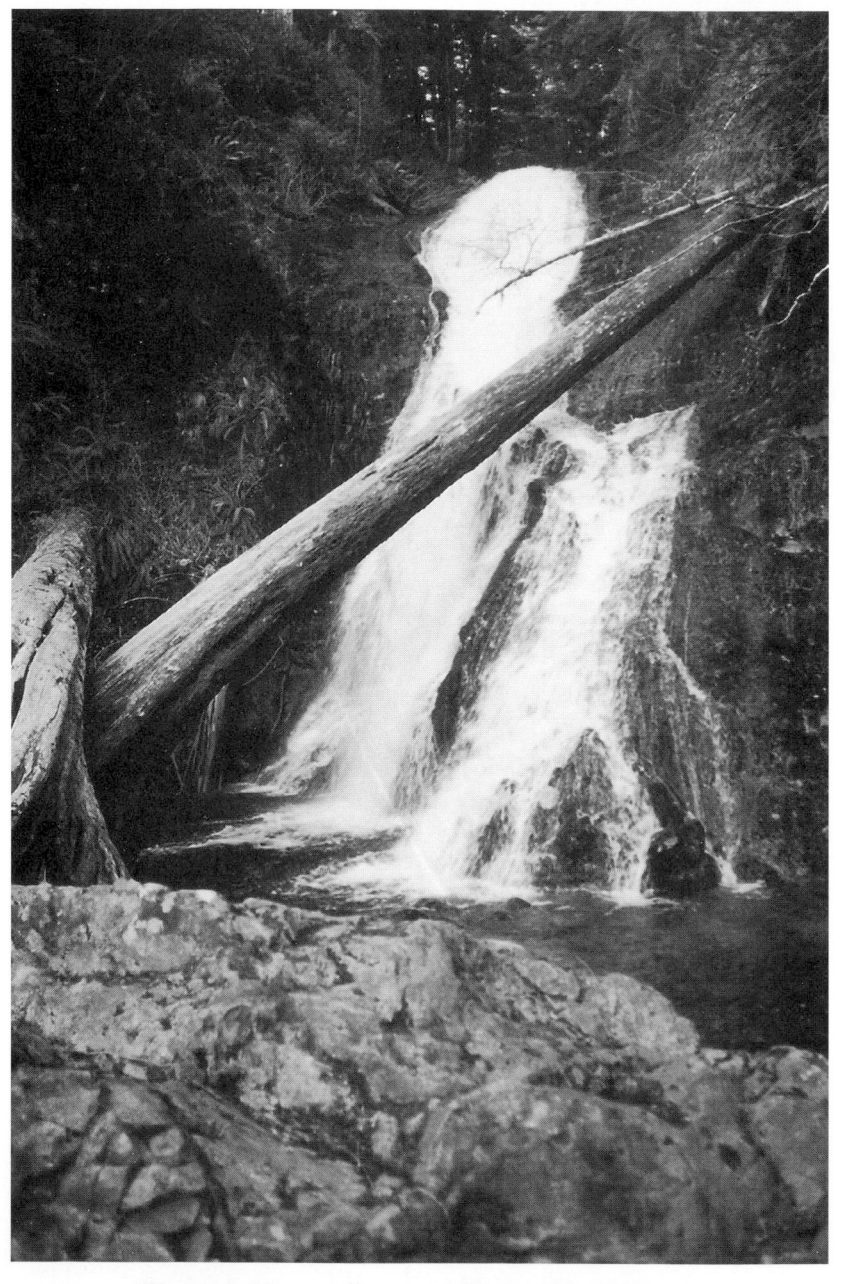

Waterfall and Pool at Pete Wolf Creek

Chapter 6
Exploring Hidden Treasures

The Juan de Fuca Marine Trail holds many secrets. Let your adventurous spirit take you to some hard-to-find destinations that you might otherwise walk past without even noticing. This chapter describes the hidden treasures, followed by descriptions of how to get to each location.

Please note that visiting *some* of these hidden treasures requires the use of old unmarked side trails and roads that **do not** belong to the Juan de Fuca Marine Trail system. Please read Chapter 5 for more information on their use before commencing your exploration.

1. WATERFALL AND POOL (AT CHINA BEACH)

Hidden Treasures:	waterfall and pool
Location:	the mouth of Pete Wolf Creek on China Beach
Total Distance:	2.0 kilometres there and back
Hiking Time:	1.5 hours
Suitable For:	beginner to expert

Start your hike from the China Beach trailhead lower parking lot, and walk the half-kilometre on the forest trail through the old-growth forest down to China Beach. Park rules prohibit camping and fires on China Beach, so use this pristine beach for day activities only. At the extreme west end of China Beach, if the tide remains below 2.5 metres, you can walk past the cliff and over to the boulder field. A small trail leads between the boulders to the **waterfall** and **pool** at the mouth of Pete Wolf Creek. *See the location of the falls on the map for the Unmarked Side Trail #1 - Mystic Beach at Km. 2.6 in Chapter 5.*

Hiking from the China Beach trailhead lower parking lot to the hidden waterfall takes approximately thirty minutes. Return the way you came.

Additional Information:
- Read Chapter 4: Options to Extend Your Trek, #1 - Jordan River Public Campground to China Beach Trailhead.

2. ROCK ARCH, CLIFFS, AND WHITE SANDS (AT KM. 2.5)

Hidden Treasures:	rock arch, cliffs, and the white sands of Mystic Beach
Location:	rock arch at the extreme west end of Mystic Beach; the cliffs at the east end of Mystic Beach at low tide
Total Distance:	7 kilometres there and back
Hiking Time:	from 2 to 3 hours (varies with distance hiked)
Suitable For:	beginner to expert

To view these treasures, begin your hike from the China Beach upper parking lot trailhead at Km. 0. It will take you approximately forty-five minutes to hike the 2.5 kilometres to **the white sands of Mystic Beach**. At low tide, explore the **cliffs** at the far east end of Mystic Beach, and the **rock arch** at the west end of the beach. Return the way you came.

Additional Information:
* Read Chapter 3: Forty-seven Kilometres of Wilderness Trekking, Part A - China Beach to Bear Beach, and Chapter 5: Unmarked Side Trail #1 - Mystic Beach at Km. 2.6.

Another Option:
* Hike west on the Juan de Fuca Marine Trail to the viewpoint at Km. 3.3. Look for the Trail access markers and information signs at McVicar Creek at the west end of Mystic Beach. The viewpoint at Km. 3.3 at the open-face cliff gives a commanding view of the Juan de Fuca Strait. Return the way you came. This option adds an hour or two kilometres to the hike.

3. ROCK ARCH, WATERFALLS , AND ARTIFACTS (AT KM. 9.6)

Hidden Treasures:	rock arch, log staircase, waterfall, creekbed, shipwreck artifacts, Rock-on-a-Pillar
Location:	rock arch at extreme east end of Bear Beach; waterfalls; log staircase at Km. 8.1; creekbed at Km. 8.6; artifacts at Km. 10.1; Rock-on-a-Pillar Km. 10.5
Total Distance:	9 kilometres there and back
Hiking Time:	from 3 to 4 hours (varies with distance hiked)
Suitable For:	intermediate to expert

To begin this hike, drive west from the China Beach turnoff for 6.6 kilometres along Highway #14 to the Clinch Creek bridge. On the east side of the Clinch Creek bridge, look for an old gated road on the south side of the highway. On the north side of the highway, look for a twenty-centimeter sign with a numeral 3 on it. Park your vehicle two or more metres off the highway, and avoid blocking access to the gated road. Commence your hike by following the old road past the gravel pit, then to the trail, down to Bear Beach. Refer to the map and directions for Unmarked Side Trail #2 - Clinch Creek at Km. 9.6 in Chapter 5.

When you arrive at the beach (Km. 9.6 on Bear Beach), proceed east to Rosemond Creek. The **high-tide beach cutoff** immediately west of Rosemond Creek becomes impassable when the tide rises above three metres. Large waves crashing on the beach may render the cutoff impassible at lower tides, too. If you can see solid ground, the cutoff remains passable. *See the photograph of this cutoff area on the colour contour map.* When you arrive at Rosemond Creek, explore up the **creek bed** if the water level is low. After heavy rains, the creek becomes very swollen, making exploring upstream impossible.

For a great view, climb the **log stairs** beside the **waterfall** at Km. 8.1 on Bear Beach. Continue walking east on the beach past the towering cliffs to the **rock arch** located at the east end.

Take the time to visit the geological wonder at the west end of the beach called **Rock-on-a-Pillar**. You will see the **artifacts** from a shipwreck at the sandy point near Km. 10. Return to your vehicle the way you came. In order to return to Highway #14, you must remember where the unmarked side trail joins the beach. Locate the unmarked side trail only thirty-five paces east of the mouth of Clinch Creek.

Additional Information:
* Read Chapter 3: Forty-seven Kilometres of Wilderness Trekking, Part B - Bear Beach to Chin Beach, and Chapter 5: Unmarked Side Trail #2 - Clinch Creek at Km. 9.6.

Another Option:
* Hike to the top of the hill at Km. 11 for a view of the Juan de Fuca Strait.

4. CREEK POOLS AND HIDDEN BEACH (AT KM. 12)

Hidden Treasures:	creek pools and hidden beach
Location:	Hoard Creek at Km. 12
Total Distance:	4 kilometres there and back
Hiking Time:	2 hours
Suitable For:	beginner to expert

To start this hike, you must first find the gated emergency road located along Highway #14. Begin by driving west for 9.2 kilometres along Highway #14 from the China Beach trailhead turnoff. On the north side of Highway #14, opposite the gated road, look for a twenty-centimeter sign with a numeral 4 on it. To avoid driving past the gated road, slow down when you reach the nine-kilometre mark on your vehicle odometer. Park your vehicle well off to the side of Highway #14 so that you will not block access to the emergency road.

You can reach the Juan de Fuca Marine Trail on a short ten-minute hike down the road. Refer to the map and directions for Unmarked Side Trail #3 - Magdalena Point at Km. 13 in Chapter 5. Take the left (east) fork of the road, and you will soon see a Juan de Fuca Marine Trail sign. Follow the Trail east to Hoard Creek. Explore the tiny **hidden beach**, and visit the **clear pools** upstream. A cleared rest area beside the bridge makes a great spot for a trail lunch. Return the way you came.

Additional Information:
- Read Chapter 3: Forty-seven Kilometres of Wilderness Trekking, Part B - Bear Beach to Chin Beach, and Chapter 5: Unmarked Side Trail #3 - Magdalena Point at Km. 13.

Other Options:
- Continue east along the trail to Bear Beach and Rock-on-a-Pillar. Be prepared to climb some very steep hills. These three kilometres will add two hours to your trek. Return the way you came.
- If you wish to embark on a wonderful two- or three-kilometre excursion through old-growth forest, follow the trail west to Magdalena Point or beyond. Return the way you came. Estimate an additional half-hour for each extra kilometre of hiking you do.

5. Giant Cedars, Beach, and Rock Arch (at Km. 21)

Hidden Treasures:	old growth cedar trees, wild beach, rock arch
Location:	the old-growth cedar trees on the Hidden Trail; the rock arch west of the #3 high-tide cutoff on Chin Beach; Emergency Shelter at Km. 20.5
Total Distance:	6 kilometres there and back
Hiking Time:	from 3 to 5 hours (varies with distance hiked)
Suitable For:	intermediate to expert

Before looking for these treasures, park a vehicle at the hidden side trail located approximately 1.7 kilometres east of the ninety-degree turn going down to Loss Creek bridge along Highway #14. Use the map and directions for the Unmarked Side Trail #4: Chin Beach at Km. 21 in Chapter 5 to find the location of the hidden side trail. Park your vehicle two or more metres off Highway #14 and commence your hike.

The two-kilometre hike to Chin Beach will take from forty to fifty minutes. *Ten minutes from Highway #14 you will pass the* **giant cedar** *pictured on the back cover of this book.*

The side trail meets Chin Beach behind the marker at Km. 21, directly east of the pit toilets and a little stream. You may want to visit the **emergency shelter** at the east end of the **beach**. To find the shelter, climb up the main trail to the bluff located at the east end of the beach.

Visit the **rock arch** at Km. 21.7 only at the full- or new-moon tides, when the tide falls below one metre. When the tide falls that low, you can walk through the rock arch and shore caves. At tides above one metre, use the forest trail at Km. 21.3 to hike around this area of the beach. Return the way you came.

Additional Information:
* Read Chapter 3: Forty-seven Kilometres of Wilderness Trekking, Part B - Chin Beach to Sombrio Beach, and Chapter 5: Unmarked Side Trail #4 - Chin Beach at Km. 21.

Another Option:
* Hike from Chin Beach to the Loss Creek bridge and back. Estimate an additional four kilometres and two hours hiking time.

6. GORGE, SEA LION CAVES AND REEF SHELF (AT KM. 25)

Hidden Treasures:	suspension bridge and gorge, sea lion caves, and reef shelf
Location:	Loss Creek suspension bridge and gorge at Trail Km. 23.8; Trail to sea lion caves at Km. 25; Sombrio Point reef shelf at Km. 26.7
Total Distance:	6 to 10 kilometres there and back
Hiking Time:	from 3 to 6 hours (varies with distance hiked)
Suitable For:	intermediate to expert (Loss Creek hike is suitable for beginners)

Find these treasures by driving west for 18.8 kilometres along Highway #14 from the China Beach trailhead turnoff, or drive two kilometres west of the Loss Creek bridge on Highway #14. Look for the yellow gate in front of the logging road on the south side of Highway #14. Watch for a twenty-centimeter sign with a numeral 7 on it located on the north side of the highway opposite the gate. Park your vehicle on the north side of the highway.

Before you start exploring these treasures, refer to the map and directions for Unmarked Side Trail #5 - Loss Creek at Km. 25.

If you are visiting the Loss Creek **suspension bridge** and **gorge**, commence your hike from Highway #14, and follow the unmarked side trail (logging road) for two kilometres. Do not take the right fork to Sombrio Point. Continue hiking past the marker for Km. 25 to the end of the road. Continue to the suspension bridge at Km. 23.8 through the forest on the Juan de Fuca Marine Trail.

If you plan to visit the **sea lion caves**, commence your hike from Highway #14, and follow the unmarked side trail (logging road) for two kilometres. Do not take the right fork to Sombrio Point. Continue hiking past the marker at Km. 25 until you reach the rusted cable lying on the road. Immediately past the cable and seventeen paces before the end of the road, look for the sea lion trail on the west side of the road. Currently, there are little stones painted white immediately in front of the sea lion trail. This hidden trail follows a steep ridge down to little islands and caves frequented by sea lions. This trail can be overgrown, rough, and dangerous where it traverses the cliffs above the sea lion caves. Enjoy observing sea lions in their natural habitat. Please be careful not to disturb the marine mammals.

If you plan to visit the **reef shelf** at Sombrio Point, commence your hike from Highway #14, and follow the unmarked side trail (logging road) for two kilometres. Take the west fork and continue to the end of the road. Follow the steep ridge trail down to Sombrio Point at Km. 26.8 to see spectacular views of Sombrio Beach. On days when the tide is low, make your way down onto the reef shelf and explore this wild shoreline.

Additional Information:
* Read Chapter 3: Forty-seven Kilometres of Wilderness Trekking, Part C - Chin Beach to Sombrio Beach, and Chapter 5: Unmarked Side Trail #5 - Loss Creek at Km. 25.

7. HIDDEN WATERFALLS AND POOLS (AT KM. 27 TO 30)

Hidden Treasures:	hidden waterfalls, pools
Location:	waterfall on Sombrio Beach at Km. 27.6; waterfall and pools above the bay at Km. 27.2
Total Distance:	6 kilometres there and back
Hiking Time:	from 3 to 4 hours (varies with distance hiked)
Suitable For:	beginner to expert

To find the hidden waterfalls and pools, drive to Sombrio Beach trailhead and start your hike from the parking lot. Follow the Juan de Fuca Marine Trail to the beach. Hike to the east end of the beach only at low tide to avoid delays at the high-tide cutoff at Km. 27.8. When you arrive at the extreme east end of Sombrio Beach, take the main Juan de Fuca Marine Trail for a short fifteen-minute hike up to the bridge and waterfall. Explore up the creek bed to see more **waterfalls** and **pools**.

Return to the beach. Find the stream just west of the pit toilets and marker ball at Km. 27.5. Follow the stream back into a gorge as far as you can for a view of the **hidden waterfall** and **pool**. If time permits, explore the beach immediately east of the Sombrio River mouth. Return the way you came.

Additional Information:
* Read Chapter 3: Forty-seven Kilometres of Wilderness Trekking, Part C - Chin Beach to Sombrio River.

Other Options:
* Follow the Juan de Fuca Marine Trail east of Sombrio Beach to Sombrio Point at Km. 26.8 for great views of the beach and the Juan de Fuca Strait. On days when the tide is low, explore the reef shelf. The waves crashing on the reef can be spectacular

during storms. Return the way you came.

- Follow Sombrio Beach west to view the high-tide cutoff. A hiking stick will make the required boulder-hopping easier. Return the way you came.

8. SEAL GROTTO, TIDE POOLS, AND FALLS (AT KM. 38)

Hidden Treasures:	seal grotto, tide pools and reef shelf, waterfalls and hidden beach
Location:	seal grotto at the mouth of Parkinson Creek; reef shelf and tide pools located between Km. 38 and Km. 39
Total Distance:	from 1 to 8 kilometres there and back
Hiking Time:	from 1 to 7 hours (varies with distance hiked)
Suitable For:	beginner to expert

The most fascinating destination on the entire Juan de Fuca Marine Trail leads to the Parkinson Creek seal grotto. This magical spot remained a secret for many years, until recently, when detailed television stories and magazine articles gave these caves extensive media coverage. A ten-minute walk from the parking lot of the Parkinson Creek trailhead brings you to the seal caves, the grotto, a birthing den, and a view of the Juan de Fuca Strait. If seals are present, please be extremely quiet so you do not disturb them. To ensure that these magnificent creatures return year-after-year, we must all respect their habitat.

To find the caves from the parking lot, where the three roads meet, walk southeastward past the information board and the double-post gate for only eighty paces to the first overgrown gravel road. Follow the overgrown gravel road directly south for another 35 paces to a little unmarked trail that leads into the underbrush off to the right. Follow the unmarked trail through the underbrush in a southwesterly direction for ten minutes until you come to a clearing just above the observation area. Before you proceed to the observation area, make your way over a fallen tree to get to the shoreline reefs for a view of the Juan de Fuca Strait. Then return to the observation area to view the **seal grotto**, near the mouth of Parkinson Creek. Return the way you came.

For another exciting view of the caves and creekbed, you can follow Parkinson Creek to its mouth. **Waterfalls** cascading down the creek make this creek bed a great place to explore. When Parkinson

Creek looks swollen because of heavy rains, postpone this adventure. Go this way only if the water level in the creek is low. First, you must get on the west side of the Parkinson Creek bridge. Cross the bridge by walking west from the parking lot for about five minutes. Follow the trail beside Parkinson Creek on the west side of the bridge for about forty metres. Find the little path that leads to the creek bed. This overgrown path takes you to the second set of pools below the bridge. Follow the creek bed downstream from the second set of pools. *Do not swim in the pools. Hikers draw their drinking water from this stream.* When you come to the impassable pool near the caves, stop, and do not try to go any farther. Otherwise, you risk falling over a fifteen-metre waterfall. You will see the **hidden beach** below the large rock arch leading to the seal caves. The view of the area from this vantage point is spectacular. *For a good grip on slippery rocks, wear reef boots or sandals when exploring streambeds. Reef boots allow you to wade in the creek. Always keep your hiking boots dry.* Return the way you came.

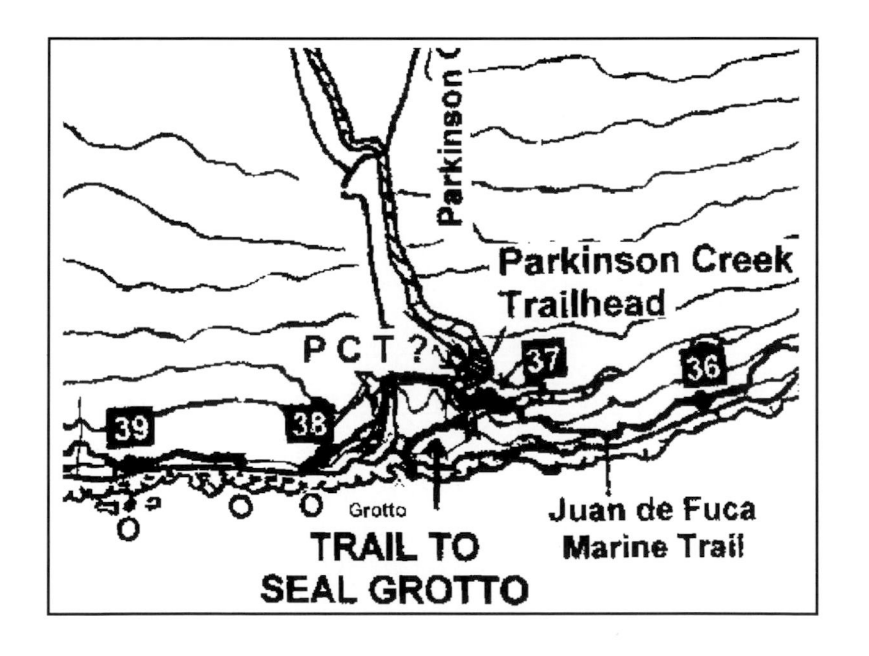

Parkinson Creek Area

Exploring the reef shelf can be exciting. Tide pools, huge waves, and scenic views of the Juan de Fuca Strait and Olympic Mountains make this a popular destination. Take this route only at very low tides. High tide will stop you at a small hidden beach just before the grotto entrance. Refer to your tide guide to find the low-tide times before starting your hike to the reef shelf. Follow the Juan de Fuca Marine Trail west past Parkinson Creek bridge and on to Km. 38, where the Trail leads onto the **reef shelf**. Follow the reef shelf eastward along the shoreline. The reef holds many large **tide pools** to view along the way. Find the small hidden beach just before the grotto entrance. At low tide, once you have passed the small beach, continue to the grotto entrance. Keep an eye on the rising tide, and return the way you came.

Additional Information:
• Read Chapter 3: Forty-seven Kilometres of Wilderness Trekking, Part D - Sombrio Beach to Parkinson Creek (last three paragraphs) and Part E - Parkinson Creek to Botanical Beach.

Another Option:
• Hike west to Providence Cove at Km. 40.6 and explore the reef shelf on your return hike back to Parkinson Creek. Take time to view the Payzant Creek waterfall, the reef shelf, and the seal grotto observation area as described above.

9. TIDE POOLS (AT KM. 46)

Hidden Treasure:	tide pools
Location:	The Shoreline Trail to Botany Bay; Botanical Beach tide pools on the reef shelf between Km. 46 and Botany Bay
Total Distance:	from 3 to 4 kilometres there and back
Hiking Time:	from 2 to 4 hours (varies with distance hiked)
Suitable For:	beginner to expert

Begin your hike to the tide pools from the Botanical Beach trailhead. High tides flood the reef, so you must plan to visit at very low tides (below 1.2 metres). Tide guide information is usually posted at trailheads on information boards. Start your hike only after you have this information. You may want to arrive at the Trail with your own Sooke Tide Guide, which you can buy at local hardware stores, fishing stores, and marinas.

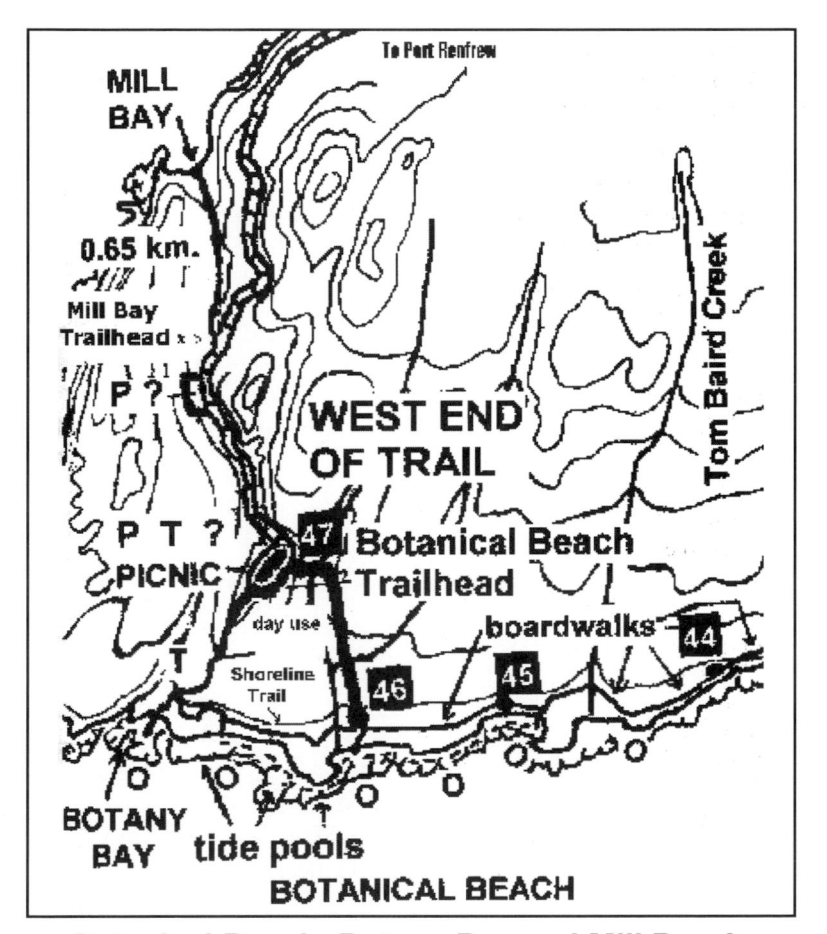

Botanical Beach, Botany Bay and Mill Bay Area

Take the wide, gentle-sloping trail at the east side of the parking lot to the beach. This one-kilometre walk, suitable for all ages, leads down to Botanical Beach. When you reach Km. 46, follow the stairs down to the beach, and continue west onto the reef shelf to view the **tide pools**.

You can also access the reef shelf by using the Shoreline Trail that is an integral part of the Botanical Beach special interest zone.

73

The trail connects Botanical Beach with Botany Bay. You can hike on this trail, which lies between Botanical Beach and Botany Bay, to the next bay and access the **tide pool reef** from there. At Km. 26, go down the stairs to find the Shoreline Trail to the main tide pool area.

Plan to visit the popular Botany Bay on the way back to the parking lot by hiking west on the Shoreline Trail from Km. 46. Botany Bay is a very beautiful and isolated beach. The trail is suitable for children and active seniors.

Additional Information:
• Read Chapter 3: Forty-seven Kilometres of Wilderness Trekking, Part E - Parkinson Creek to Botanical Beach.

Another Option:
• Hike west on the Juan de Fuca Marine Trail to Km. 44.5, and view the rock island, along with reef pools and surge channels carved into the rocky shore. Visit the tide pools and reef shelf at low tide. Return the way you came. This would add three kilometres and approximately two hours to the hike.

10. SECLUDED BEACH AND WATERFALLS (AT MILL BAY)

Hidden Treasures:	secluded beach, waterfalls hidden in the forest
Location:	Mill Bay Beach Trail
Total Distance:	1.3 kilometres there and back
Hiking Time:	from 40 to 60 minutes
Suitable For:	beginner to expert

To reach the secluded beach and waterfalls, you can start your trek from the Mill Bay trailhead parking lot located one kilometre north of the Botanical Beach parking lot. Mill Bay, a secluded beach on the shores of Port San Juan, got its name from the sawmill built there in 1880. Be sure to read the history of this beach on the information board at the Mill Bay trailhead. Your hike from the parking lot to the **secluded beach** takes you past **hidden waterfalls**, old wooden culverts, and other artifacts. The overgrown road now looks more like a cart path. Mill Bay is for day-use hiking only. Do not camp overnight or light beach fires. Return the way you came.

The hidden treasures outlined in this chapter can be included in longer day hikes, overnight hikes, and the forty-seven-kilometre trek. Make a note on your map of the location of these extraordinary places so you can visit some of them on your next hike.

Chapter 7
Day-Hiking the Juan de Fuca
Marine Trail

The Juan de Fuca Marine Trail is ideal for day hikes. With the use of the four trailheads and the five unmarked side trails as entry and exit points, you can plan one-way day hikes on any section of the forty-seven-kilometre hike. You may even want to day hike the entire trail while staying at a Bed & Breakfast or in your camper. Please remember that the old unmarked side trails and roads **do not** belong to the Juan de Fuca Marine Trail system. Please read Chapter 5 for more information on their use before commencing your day hike.

One-way day hikes require a vehicle parked at the final destination. Before your hike, arrange to take two vehicles to the end-point of your hike. Leave one vehicle parked well off the highway and return in the second vehicle to the start point of your hike. If you only have one vehicle, arrange to drop the vehicle at the end-point of your hike and have a friend drive you to the start point of your hike. Alternatively, arrange for drop off and pick up transportation through one of the services listed in the Appendix.

Plot the unmarked side trails on your colour contour map, using the maps and directions provided in *Chapter 5: Unmarked Side Trails*. You will soon see the many possibilities for day and overnight hikes, so you can plan your own hikes. Consider the numerous examples of one-way hikes provided here. Each day-hike example details the total distance, hiking time, type of hike, and difficulty rating. You can also do most of these hikes in the opposite direction.

Hikers who want to explore hidden treasures along the trail can find them described in *Chapter 6: Exploring Hidden Treasures*. Decide on the section of trail that you want to hike, and then discover interesting things to see along the way.

For more details on the section you plan to hike, read *Chapter 3: Forty-seven Kilometres of Wilderness Trekking*.

You will find more than twenty different day hikes to enjoy on the Juan de Fuca Marine Trail. As many options exist for overnight and weekend hikes, too.

PREPARING FOR YOUR DAY HIKE

Those new to hiking should not attempt an intermediate hike unless accompanied by an experienced hiker. Be prepared, and avoid going beyond your limits. Instead of bringing alcohol or drugs on a hike, save the partying for when you get home. Return home a hiking success story, not a hiking casualty.

Begin your hike early. Start a six-hour hike between 7:00 A.M. and 9:00 A.M., not at 12:00 Noon or later. Plan to have extra daylight time in case your hike takes longer than expected.

Advise a friend or family member where and when you plan to hike. Arrange with your family to send out a search party if you do not return from your hike at the predetermined time. You may want to phone home from the nearest pay phone soon after you exit the trail.

Wear a good pair of hiking boots. Wear gaiters to keep mud, dust, and water out of your boots. If you do not own gaiters, use a pair of old socks with the soles cut off. Wear two pairs of socks, a light inner polypropylene pair and a heavier outer wool pair. Wool keeps the feet dry by drawing moisture away from the skin. The feet then become less prone to blisters caused by moisture and friction.

Heavy rains render most creeks swollen and fast-flowing. Bring reef boots, old running shoes, or sandals for quickly crossing small creeks lacking bridges. Use a pole or walking stick for balance.

Dress according to the temperature, and layer your clothing (T-shirt, shirt, fleece jacket, shorts, a hat, light wind pants, and rain gear if necessary). Avoid overheating, and avoid being chilled. You may want to wear biking gloves to protect the palms of your hands from falls and splinters. Carry a small first-aid kit that includes blister pads, moleskin, tweezers, iodine, rubbing alcohol, bandages, and antibacterial cream.

Take enough food to last for a day and a half. Have extra food and water waiting in the car for after the hike. Take high-energy foods, including sandwiches, energy bars, trail mix, apples, oranges, and granola bars. Carry your food, water, and extra clothing in a small daypack or waist pack.

Carry a whistle, bear bells, matches, fire starter, miniature flashlight, knife, sunglasses, emergency space blanket, light gloves, this book, and the colour contour map.

The suggested day hikes, listed in topographical (the east end of the Juan de Fuca Marine Trail and conti to Botanical Beach. Some of the day hikes require the side trails, so you may need to refer to Chapter 5 for m where the side trail fits into the day hike.

1. JORDAN RIVER CAMPGROUND TO CHINA BEACH TRAILHEAD

Total Distance:	4 kilometres
Hiking Time:	from 2 to 3 hours
Type of Hike:	easy, day hike on the beach
Difficulty Rating:	for beginners to experts

This hike features a pleasant beach walk. Park a vehicle at the China Beach trailhead lower parking lot. Then arrange transportation to the Jordan River public campground, located beside the Jordan River bridge. Begin your hike by crossing the Jordan River bridge, and walk west on Highway #14 for about a hundred metres. Take the path leading down to the beach. When the high tide rises above three metres, you will have difficulty hiking on China Beach because the tide floods the beach.

Enjoy a leisurely trek, and when you arrive near the west end of the beach, find the pit toilets that mark where the trail leads up into the forest. It will take fifteen minutes to hike the half-kilometre from the beach to the lower China Beach parking lot. Hiking the entire four kilometres will take approximately an hour and a half to two hours.

Additional Information:
- See Chapter 6: Exploring Hidden Treasures, #1 - Hidden Waterfall and Pool (at China Beach).

2. MYSTIC BEACH LOOP

Total Distance:	3 kilometres
Hiking Time:	from 1.5 to 2 hours
Type of Hike:	easy, short day-hike
Difficulty Rating:	for beginners to experts

This short hike includes both forest and beach. Before starting this hike, park a vehicle at the McVicar Creek bridge. Park your vehicle two or more metres off the highway. Then walk (if using only one vehicle) or drive a second vehicle to the China Beach upper ng lot. Start your hike from the upper parking lot at the Juan de uca Marine Trail trailhead at China Beach. Follow the Juan de Fuca Marine Trail 2.5 kilometres to Mystic Beach.

At low tide, you can explore the cliffs at the far east side of the beach. You can also view and explore around the rock arch at the extreme west end of Mystic Beach. Pack a picnic lunch and enjoy the soft, sandy beach.

Locate the unmarked side trail 60 paces east of the McVicar Creek, and hike directly up to the McVicar Creek bridge on Highway #14. To find the unmarked side trail, use the map and directions in Chapter 5: Unmarked Side Trail #1 - Mystic Beach at Km. 2.6.

Additional Information:
* See Chapter 3: Forty-seven Kilometres of Wilderness Trekking, Part A - China Beach to Bear Beach, and Chapter 6: Exploring Hidden Treasures, #2 - Rock Arch, Cliffs, White Sands (at Km. 2.5).

Other Options:
* Park your car at the China Beach trailhead, hike to Mystic Beach, and return the same way to the China Beach trailhead. Allow 2.5 to 3 hours for this five to six kilometre hike.

* Park your car at McVicar Creek bridge, and hike directly to Mystic Beach on the hidden side trail located fifteen metres east of the bridge. Return the way you came. Allow one to two hours for this three-kilometre hike.

* Hike from Jordan River along China Beach and up to the China Beach trailhead, then to Mystic Beach. End your hike at the McVicar Creek bridge on Highway #14, or at the China Beach trailhead. Allow four to five hours for this seven to nine kilometre hike.

3. CHINA BEACH AT KM. 0 TO BEAR BEACH AT KM. 9.7

Total Distance:	11 kilometres
Hiking Time:	from 4 to 5 hours
Type of Hike:	intermediate, long day-hike
Difficulty Rating:	for intermediate to expert hikers
High-tide Cutoff:	Km. 8.7 on Bear Beach (above 3 metres)

Before you start this full-day hike, check your tide tables closely. You need to arrive at Bear Beach at low tide to avoid delays at the high-tide cutoff at Km. 8.7. Begin by parking a vehicle at the gated road located between Rosemond Creek and Clinch Creek. To get to this gated road, drive 6.6 kilometres west from the China Beach trailhead turnoff on Highway #14. Park your vehicle two or more metres off the highway, and avoid blocking access to the gated road. Return in a second vehicle to the China Beach trailhead to commence your hike.

Start your hike from the trailhead at the upper China Beach parking lot. Follow the Juan de Fuca Marine Trail to Mystic Beach. Look for the Trail access markers and information signs at McVicar Creek on the west end of Mystic Beach. Continue into the forest from the west end and hike to Clinch Creek on Bear Beach.

When you reach Bear Beach, continue hiking west on the beach past the high-tide cutoff located immediately west of Rosemond Creek. After heavy rains, you may have to use logs to cross the creek. Farther on, locate the unmarked side trail 35 paces east of Clinch Creek. To find the unmarked side trail, use the map and directions in Chapter 5: Unmarked Side Trail #2 - Clinch Creek at Km. 9.6. The hike from the mouth of Clinch Creek to Highway #14 will take approximately twenty minutes.

Additional Information:

*   See Chapter 3: Forty-seven Kilometres of Wilderness Trekking, Part A - China Beach to Bear Beach. Also see Chapter 6: Exploring Hidden Treasures, #2 - Rock Arch, Cliffs, White Sands (at Km. 2.5), and #3 - Rock Arch, Waterfalls and Artifacts at Km 9.6).

Another Option

*   Begin your hike from McVicar Creek bridge on Highway #14, and hike down to Mystic Beach on the unmarked side trail. From

Mystic Beach, hike the Juan de Fuca Marine Trail to Clinch Creek on Bear Beach. Hike to Highway #14 using the #2 unmarked side trail described in Chapter 5. Allow four to six hours for this nine-kilometre hike.

4. BEAR BEACH AT KM. 9.6 TO MAGDALENA POINT ROAD AT KM. 13

Total Distance:	6 kilometres
Hiking Time:	from 2 to 3 hours
Type of Hike:	hilly, difficult section, short day-hike
Difficulty Rating:	for intermediate to expert hikers

This hike would be a good one to choose if you want to include a picnic on the beach. Begin by parking a vehicle at the gated road located just past Hoard Creek. To get to this gated road, drive west for 9.2 kilometres from the China Beach trailhead turnoff on Highway #14. Park your vehicle two or more metres off the highway, and avoid blocking access to the gated road. Return in a second vehicle to the gated road just east of Clinch Creek to commence your hike.

Start your hike at the gated road just east of Clinch Creek. Use the map and directions for the Unmarked Side Trail #2: Clinch Creek at Km. 9.6, in Chapter 5. Hike down to Bear Beach and continue in a westerly direction to the end of the beach. Find the continuation of the Juan de Fuca Marine Trail at Ledingham Creek, and hike to Km. 13. You will see an old logging road from the Trail. Get onto the road and hike up to Highway #14. Just follow the road north using the map and directions in Chapter 5 for the Unmarked Side Trail #3 - Magdalena Point at Km. 13.

Additional Information:
- See Chapter 3: Forty-seven Kilometres of Wilderness Trekking, Part B - Bear Beach to Chin Beach. Also see Chapter 6: Exploring Hidden Treasures, #3 - Rock Arch, Waterfalls and Artifacts at Km 9.6) and #4 - Creek Pools and Hidden Beach (at Km. 12).

Other Options:
- Hike from Bear Beach to Chin Beach. Allow six to seven hours for this fourteen to fifteen kilometre hike. Before commencing your hike, park a vehicle at the hidden side trail located approximately 1.7 kilometres east of the ninety-degree turn going

down to Loss Creek bridge along Highway #14. Use the map and directions for the Unmarked Side Trail #4: Chin Beach at Km. 21 in Chapter 5 to find the location of the hidden side trail. Park your vehicle two or more metres off the highway. Return in a second vehicle to the gated road just east of Clinch Creek to commence your hike. Hike from Bear Beach to Chin Beach. To exit the Trail at Chin Beach, use the map and directions for the Unmarked Side Trail #4: Chin Beach at Km. 21 in Chapter 5.

• Hike from Bear Beach to Loss Creek Road at Km. 25, then on to Highway #14 using the Loss Creek Road. This eighteen-kilometre, nine-hour marathon hike is for super-athletic expert hikers only. Before commencing your hike, park a vehicle at the gated logging road two kilometres west of the Loss Creek Bridge on Highway #14. Park your vehicle on the north side of the highway opposite the gate. Return in a second vehicle to the gated road just east of Clinch Creek to commence your hike. Hike from Bear Beach to Loss Creek Road. To exit the Trail at Loss Creek Road, use the map and directions for the Unmarked Side Trail #5: Loss Creek at Km. 25 in Chapter 5.

• Super-athletic expert hikers could day-hike from Bear Beach to Sombrio Beach. Take ski poles and start at dawn for twenty kilometres of serious day hiking. This ten-hour marathon hike is for exceptionally fit hikers only. Before commencing your hike, park a vehicle at the Sombrio Beach trailhead parking lot. Return in a second vehicle to the gated road just east of Clinch Creek to commence your hike. Use the map and directions for the Unmarked Side Trail #2: Clinch Creek at Km. 9.6, in Chapter 5. Hike from Bear Beach to Sombrio Beach, exiting at the Sombrio Beach trailhead.

5. MAGDALENA POINT ROAD AT KM. 13 TO CHIN BEACH AT KM. 21

Total Distance:	11 kilometres
Hiking Time:	from 5 or 6 hours
Type of Hike:	long day-hike, some difficult hiking
Difficulty Rating:	for intermediate to expert hikers

This day-hike brings you to a pleasant beach and past giant cedars trees. Before you start your hike, park a vehicle at the hidden

81

side trail located approximately 1.7 kilometres east of the ninety-degree turn going down to Loss Creek bridge along Highway #14. Use the map and directions for the Unmarked Side Trail #4: Chin Beach at Km. 21 in Chapter 5 to find the location of the hidden side trail. Park your vehicle well off the highway. Return in a second vehicle to the gated road two kilometres west of Clinch Creek to commence your hike.

Start your hike using the map and directions in Chapter 5 for the Unmarked Side Trail #3 - Magdalena Point at Km. 13. Hike down the old road and take the right (west) fork. Halfway down this fork you will spot a Juan de Fuca Marine Trail sign.

Get onto the Trail and hike west to Chin Beach, past the emergency shelter, and onto the beach. To exit Chin Beach, locate the hidden trail that takes you back up to Highway #14. Just east of the pit toilets and stream, under a tree, look for the marker at Km. 21. Walk through the campsite located there, and find the trail that leads up into the forest.

The steep lower part of the two-kilometre-long trail can become muddy. The first kilometre climbs uphill. The second kilometre levels out and you will pass two giant cedars on your way to Highway #14. Many other old cedars stand in the forest in this area. Continue your hike back to your vehicle. To keep on track, read the map and directions in Chapter 5 for the Unmarked Side Trail #4 - Chin Beach at Km. 21.

Additional Information:
- See Chapter 3: Forty-seven Kilometres of Wilderness Trekking, Part B - Bear Beach to Chin Beach, and Chapter 6: Exploring Hidden Treasures, #5 - Giant Cedars, Beach and Rock Arch (at Km. 21).

Other Options:
- Hike from Km. 13 to Km. 25 (on the Loss Creek Road). Allow five to seven hours for this fifteen-kilometre hike. Before commencing your hike, park a vehicle at the gated logging road two kilometres west of the Loss Creek Bridge on Highway #14. Park your vehicle on the north side of the highway opposite the gate. Return in a second vehicle to the gated road at Unmarked Side Trail #3: Magdalena Point at Km. 13 as described in Chapter 5: Unmarked Side Trails. When you reach Km. 13 on the Juan de

Fuca Marine Trail, hike west to Km. 25. To exit the Trail at Loss Creek Road, use the map and directions for the Unmarked Side Trail #5: Loss Creek at Km. 25 in Chapter 5.

• Hike from Km. 13 to Sombrio Beach. This seventeen-kilometre hike takes expert hikers eight to ten hours to complete. Before commencing your hike, park a vehicle at the Sombrio Beach trailhead parking lot. Return in a second vehicle to the gated road at Unmarked Side Trail #3: Magdalena Point at Km. 13 as described in Chapter 5: Unmarked Side Trails. When you reach Km. 13 on the Juan de Fuca Marine Trail, hike west to Sombrio Beach, exiting at the Sombrio Beach trailhead.

6. CHIN BEACH AT KM. 21 TO LOSS CREEK ROAD AT KM. 25

Total Distance:	8 kilometres
Hiking Time:	from 3 to 5 hours
Type of Hike:	long day-hike, intermediate sections
Difficulty Rating:	for intermediate to expert hikers
High-tide Cutoff:	From Km. 21.5 to Km. 22, stay off the beach and use the forest trail.

This hike takes you through old-growth forests, onto pristine beaches and over deep gorges. Before commencing your hike, park a vehicle at the Loss Creek logging road located two kilometres west of the Loss Creek bridge on Highway #14. Park your vehicle on the north side of the highway opposite the gate. Get a ride, or return in a second vehicle to the hidden side trail approximately 1.7 kilometres east of the ninety-degree turn going down to Loss Creek bridge along Highway #14. This hidden trail is difficult to find. Use the map and directions for the Unmarked Side Trail #4 - Chin Beach at Km. 21 in Chapter 5 to locate the hidden side trail.

Hike down the hidden trail to Chin Beach at Km. 21. Commence hiking westward on the beach to Km. 21.5, and take the forest trail at the rocky point. The tide usually blocks the beach route west of the marker ball. Use the forest route.

When you reach the trail marker at Km. 25 on Loss Creek Road, continue your hike back to your vehicle using the map and directions in Chapter 5 for the Unmarked Side Trail #5 - Loss Creek at Km. 25.

Additional Information:
- See Chapter 3: Forty-seven Kilometres of Wilderness Trekking, Part C - Chin Beach to Sombrio Beach, and Chapter 6: Exploring Hidden Treasures, #6 - Gorge, Sea Lion Caves and Reef Shelf (at Km. 25).

Another Option:
- Hike from Chin Beach to Sombrio River. Allow four to six hours for this ten-kilometre hike. Before commencing your hike, park a vehicle at the Sombrio Beach trailhead parking lot. Get a ride, or return in a second vehicle to the hidden side trail located approximately 1.7 kilometres east of the ninety-degree turn going down to Loss Creek bridge along Highway #14. This hidden trail is difficult to find Use the map and directions for the Unmarked Side Trail #4 - Chin Beach at Km. 21 in Chapter 5 to locate the hidden side trail. Use the hidden side trail to access Chin Beach. Hike west from Km. 21 to Sombrio Beach, exiting at the Sombrio Beach trailhead.

7. LOSS CREEK ROAD AT KM. 25 TO SOMBRIO RIVER AT KM. 28.7

Total Distance:	6 kilometres
Hiking Time:	from 4 to 5 hours
Type of Hike:	short day-hike, some difficult sections
Difficulty Rating:	for intermediate to expert hikers
High-tide Cutoff:	Sombrio Beach at Km. 27.8

This day-hike brings you along an old logging trail as well as through both forest and beach scenery. Before commencing your hike, park a vehicle at the Sombrio Beach trailhead parking lot. Get transportation back to Loss Creek road by using a second vehicle, or get a friend to drive you. Locate Loss Creek logging road two kilometres east of the Sombrio Beach access on Highway #14. On the north side of the road opposite the yellow gate, you will see a twenty-centimeter sign with the numeral 7 on it. Park on the north side of Highway #14.

You can start your hike by using the map and directions in Chapter 5 for the Unmarked Side Trail #5: Loss Creek at Km. 25. Hike down the old logging road to the fork, and follow the Juan de Fuca Marine Trail west to Sombrio Point, then to Sombrio Beach. If time permits, be sure to explore the hidden treasures (see Additional Information below).

Be careful as you proceed along the cliff from Sombrio Point to the beach, because the trail can be very slippery. Take your time and enjoy the spectacular views.

Additional Information:
- See Chapter 3: Forty-seven Kilometres of Wilderness Trekking, Part C - Chin Beach to Sombrio Beach, and Chapter 6: Exploring Hidden Treasures, #7 - Hidden Waterfalls and Pools (at Km. 27 to 30).

Another Option:
- Hike from Loss Creek road to Parkinson Creek. These fourteen kilometres will take at least five to six hours to hike. This hike is suitable for athletic experienced hikers. Before commencing your hike, park a vehicle at the Parkinson Creek trailhead parking lot. Get a ride, or return in a second vehicle to Loss Creek road. Locate Loss Creek logging road two kilometres east of the Sombrio Beach access on Highway #14. On the north side of the road opposite the yellow gate, you will see a twenty-centimeter sign with the numeral 7 on it. Park on the north side of Highway #14. Using the map and directions in Chapter 5 for the Unmarked Side Trail #5: Loss Creek at Km. 25, hike west from Km. 25 to Parkinson Creek. Exit at the Parkinson Creek trailhead.

8. SOMBRIO BEACH AT KM. 29 TO PARKINSON CREEK AT KM. 37.2

Total Distance:	8.5 kilometres
Hiking Time:	from 3 to 5 hours
Type of Hike:	long, rough day-hike, on winding, uneven trail
Difficulty Rating:	for intermediate to expert hikers

On this hike, you can include a stop at some of the hidden treasures of the Juan de Fuca Marine Trail. Before commencing your hike, park a vehicle at Parkinson Creek trailhead parking lot. Arrange transportation, or use a second vehicle to return to the Sombrio Beach trailhead.

Start your hike from the Sombrio Beach trailhead parking lot, walk across the suspension bridge, and hike westward down to the beach. Continue hiking west on the beach past the high-tide cutoff and to the forest trail at Km. 30. Here a beach marker ball hangs in a tree, and an information board with maps gives you a general idea of the Trail.

Stop and enjoy the waterfall at Minute Creek gorge and the Thunder Rock Blowhole at Km. 32.4 on your way to Parkinson Creek trailhead. Be sure to check the additional information below if you want to explore before you drive home.

Additional Information:
See Chapter 3: Forty-seven Kilometres of Wilderness Trekking, Part D - Sombrio Beach to Parkinson Creek. Also see #7 - Hidden Waterfalls and Pools (at Km. 27 to 30), and #9 - Seal Grotto, Tide Pools, and Falls (at Km. 38) in Chapter 6: Exploring Hidden Treasures.

Another Option:
• If you want to expend some energy, start very early and hike the 18.5 kilometres from Sombrio Beach trailhead to Botanical Beach trailhead. This hike is definitely for advanced, expert hikers only. Pick a sunny day. Park your car at Botanical Beach, and arrange transportation, or have a friend drive you to Sombrio Beach, where you will start your day trek. The 18.5-kilometre hike will take eight to ten hours. You will sleep soundly after this! Wear bells, take plenty of high-energy food, and drink at least four litres of water during your hike. When you get off the trail at Botanical Beach, drive to Port Renfrew and telephone home to let your family or friends know you made it safely off the trail.

9.   PARKINSON CREEK AT KM. 37.2 TO BOTANICAL BEACH AT KM. 47

Total Distance:	10 kilometres
Hiking Time:	from 3 to 4 hours for advanced hikers, 6 hours for slow hikers
Type of Hike:	long day-hike
Difficulty Rating:	for intermediate to expert hikers

This popular day-hike could include exploring the mystical Parkinson Creek seal grotto and the famous Botanical Beach tide pools. Before commencing your hike, park a vehicle at the Botanical Beach trailhead parking lot. Then drive a second vehicle or get a ride to Parkinson Creek trailhead parking lot, where you will start your hike.

Commence hiking in a westerly direction to the Parkinson Creek bridge. Check the additional information and options below to ensure that you allow extra time for exploring. Follow the Juan de Fuca Marine Trail signs to the forest trail. Hike to Botanical Beach, where you can take the opportunity to view the tide pools at tides below 1.2 metres. End your trek by hiking up to the Botanical Beach parking lot to your vehicle.

Additional Information:
- See Chapter 3: Forty-seven Kilometres of Wilderness Trekking, Part E - Parkinson Creek to Botanical Beach, Chapter 4: #2 - Botany Bay/Botanical Beach Trail Loop; and Chapter 6: Exploring Hidden Treasures, #9 - Seal Grotto, Tide Pools, and Falls (at Km. 38).

Other Options:
- At Botanical Beach, visit the tide pools and hike the Shoreline Trail described in Chapter 6: Exploring Hidden Treasures, #9 - Tide Pools (at Km. 46).

- Before leaving the Botanical Beach parking lot, visit the Mill Bay day-use area. See Chapter 6: Exploring Hidden Treasures, #10 - Secluded Beach and Waterfalls (at Mill Bay).

WHAT COULD BE BETTER?

Day hiking can be lots of fun for those who lack the experience and equipment to partake of overnight hikes. Short hikes allow you to travel light, explore more, and hike farther than backpackers carrying a heavy pack. Once you become familiar with the Juan de Fuca Marine Trail on day hikes, you may decide to plan overnight backpacking trips to sleep under the stars. Chapter 8 outlines some of the many possibilities open to hikers who want to enjoy overnight backpacking trips and experience an evening in the wilderness with friends beside a cozy campfire.

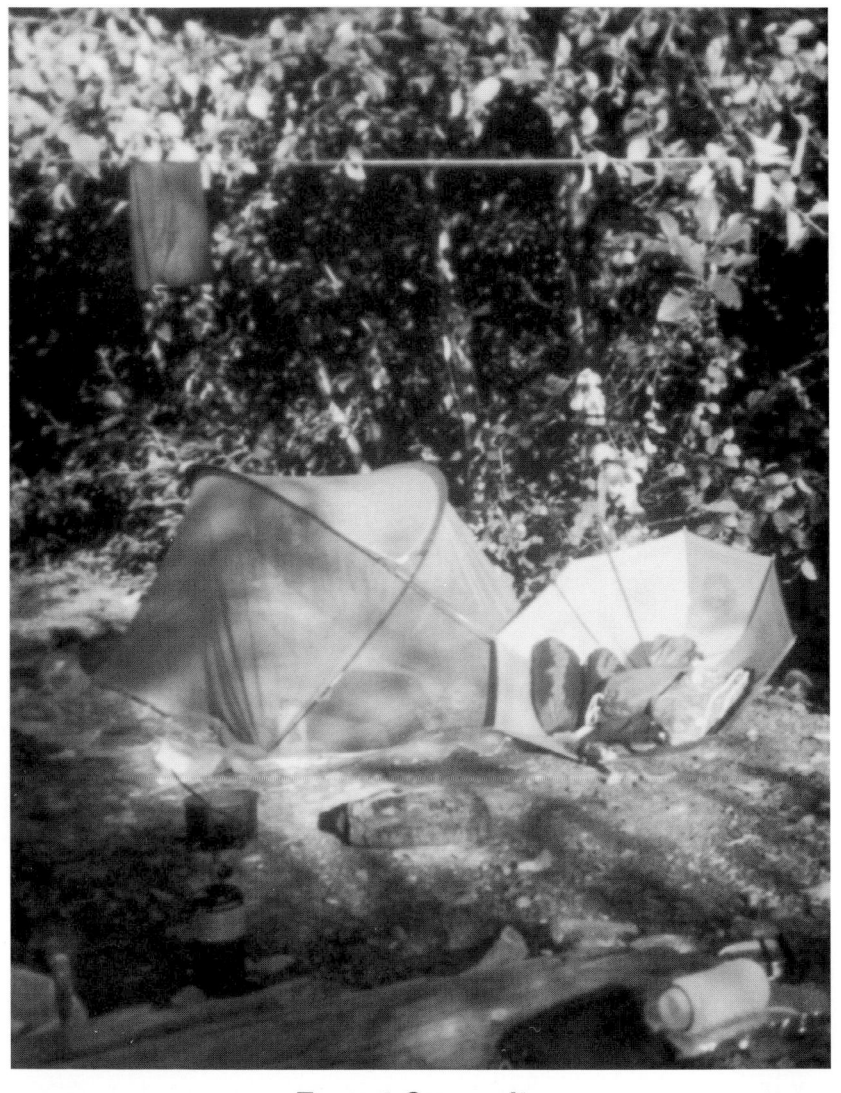

Forest Campsite

Chapter 8
Weekend Overnight Backpacking

Many hiking trails close to civilization on South Vancouver Island offer day hiking only. The isolated but easily accessible Juan de Fuca Marine Trail offers overnight camping as well as day hiking. In addition, it gives hikers the experience of being in the wilderness and beside the ocean. Numerous possibilities await hikers for weekend or mid-week overnight backpacking on the Juan de Fuca Marine Trail. You can choose from many exciting one-night trips or plan longer two-night or three-night excursions.

The first seven chapters of *Giant Cedars, White Sands* organize and present every aspect of the Trail. Chapter 8 will help you select possible routes for overnight backpacking trips. Prepare yourself by reading the previous chapters for a better idea of where, on the Trail, you would like to hike. Bring your trail book and map, keep them handy in your pack for reference on your hike, and obtain a current tide guide specifically for the Sooke area.

The length and difficulty of your hike depends on the entry and exit points of your trek. The five unmarked side trails on the maps in Chapter 5 will help you get an overall picture of the trail and its potential. Note the wilderness campground locations at Jordan River public campground, Mystic Beach, Bear Beach, Chin Beach, Sombrio Beach, Little Kuitsche Creek, and Payzant Creek. Make a note of the location of the four trailheads, already well marked on the map. By using your map in this way, you can plan hikes of almost any distance and choose the type of terrain you want to hike.

Before your hike, stop at one of the four main trailheads and deposit the required overnight camping fee into the red deposit box. Please read the rules regarding camping and fees on the information board.

Novice hikers can start with short hikes and gradually work their way up to short backpacking trips. More experienced trekkers might want to combine the Juan de Fuca Marine Trail with the West Coast Trail into one grand super-trek.

If you want to arrange transportation to and from Victoria or between different trailheads, see the listings in the Appendix, or phone a tourist information center for the staff's recommendations.

Do not start campfires at the forest campsites. If you want a campfire, plan to camp on Sombrio, Chin, Bear, or Mystic Beach. Before your hike, park a vehicle at your final hiking destination. Then use a second vehicle, or have a friend drive you to the starting point of your overnight hike. Do not rush your trek. If you arrange to meet someone to pick you up at your final destination, you may want to set a time that will allow you to do some exploring.

Be adventurous, and plan your own overnight hikes. The following examples of overnight trips will start you thinking.

1. CHINA BEACH TRAILHEAD TO MYSTIC BEACH: 5 KILOMETRES (FIRST-TIME TREKKERS)

Novice backpackers may want to begin by planning a simple overnight or weekend hike to Mystic Beach from the China Beach trailhead. You can find more information about this area in Chapter 7: Day-hiking the Juan de Fuca Marine Trail, #2 - Mystic Beach Loop. Before you know it, your thirst for bigger adventures will take hold.

2. CHINA BEACH TRAILHEAD TO BEAR BEACH: 11 KILOMETRES (FIRST-TIME TREKKERS)

Novice hikers may attempt this trip after gaining a sense of the forest through day hiking. Practice by carrying a full pack on day hikes. Before you plan this trip, read Chapter 7: Day-hiking the Juan de Fuca Marine Trail, #3 - China Beach at Km. 0 to Bear Beach at Km. 9.7 for more details about this section of the Trail.

3. JORDAN RIVER TO BEAR BEACH: 15 KILOMETRES

All levels of hikers will enjoy this beach-oriented hike. Three beaches and several kilometres of forest hiking make this hike an ideal weekend for novice hikers accompanied by more experienced hikers. Combine the following two day-hikes, detailed in Chapter 7: Day-hiking the Juan de Fuca Marine Trail:

- #1 - Jordan River Campground to China Beach Trailhead via China Beach, and
- #3 - China Beach at Km. 0 to Bear Beach at Km. 9.7.

Camp on Mystic Beach or Bear Beach.

4. MAGDALENA POINT TO SOMBRIO BEACH: 17 KILOMETRES

Intermediate and advanced hikers will enjoy the challenges on this section of the trail. This hike is a combination of three different day-hikes. To find full details, read the following sections of Chapter 7: Day-hiking the Juan de Fuca Marine Trail:

- #5 - Magdalena Point Road at Km. 13 to Chin Beach at Km. 21,
- #6 - Chin Beach at Km. 21 to Loss Creek Road at Km. 25, and
- #7 - Loss Creek Road at Km. 25 to Sombrio River at Km. 28.7.

Camp at Chin Beach. Use the Emergency Shelter at Chin Beach if inclement weather rolls in.

5. LOSS CREEK ROAD TO PARKINSON CREEK: 14 KILOMETRES

Hikers getting a late start will want to choose an option that will allow them to hike, yet give them an evening by a campfire on the beach. Combine the following two day-hikes detailed in Chapter 7: Day-hiking the Juan de Fuca Marine Trail:

- #7 - Loss Creek Road at Km. 25 to Sombrio River at Km. 28.7, and
- #8 - Sombrio Beach at Km. 29 to Parkinson Creek at Km. 37.2.

You may want to camp at Sombrio Beach the first night and then spend the next day exploring. You can also camp in the forest at the Little Kuitsche Creek campground. Use your stove when camping in the forest. If you want a campfire, plan to camp on Sombrio Beach. If you plan to explore the Parkinson Creek area, see Chapter 6: Exploring Hidden Treasures, #8 - Seal Grotto, Tide Pools, and Falls (at Km. 38) for more information.

Now that you have some examples of how to use the Juan de Fuca Marine Trail, you can expand upon these ideas and plan your own hikes. Use the descriptions in the preceding chapters to get a general idea of the attractions and sights you want to see.

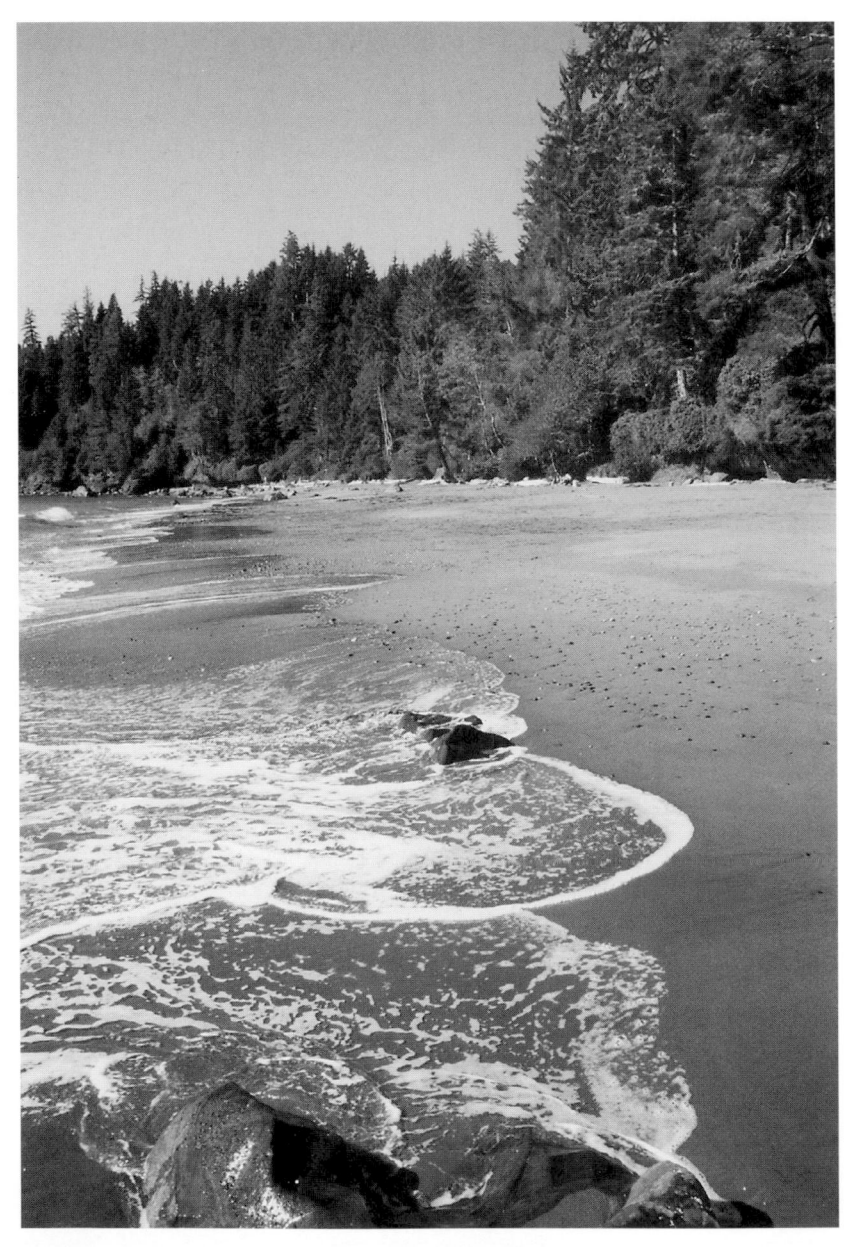

Mystic Beach

Chapter 9
Higher Places

What is so appealing about hiking in the forest? Everything in the forest contributes to a feeling of total freedom and peacefulness. Could there be more to the forest than we see or otherwise normally sense? The answer depends on our awareness.

Start with yourself, and become aware of your own internal rhythm. Your breathing and your heartbeat keep you alive with their unceasing rhythm. Natural rhythms in nature include ocean waves, tides rising and falling, changing seasons, and much more. The whole universe (existence) has rhythm.

Observe the ocean waves crashing on the beach. You may want to try breathing with this ebb and flow of the ocean waves. As the waves crash on the shore, breathe in the energy released by the crashing waves. As a wave runs back into the ocean, breathe out. See whether every seventh wave is bigger than the previous six waves. If you concentrate on the wind, you will realize that it blows in waves, too. Give it your full, undivided attention.

The babbling brook also has a rhythm. The sound of the water permeates the area of the forest immediately surrounding the stream. Naturalists have recorded the sound of babbling brooks and sold these on cassette tapes to nature-hungry city dwellers. They are trying to bring the forest to the people.

Focus your attention on birdcalls. Listening becomes more exciting if you use a pair of binoculars to spot the birds that do the singing. As you listen to the birds, feel the depth of their calls as they come from every direction. Your ears may tune in to the locations of the birds if you concentrate on their songs. Listen for different species, and make a mental note of the number of different species of birds you might be hearing.

To gain an appreciation of wherever you are take a minute or two to sense all that you can around you. In time, without having to think about doing it, you will automatically focus your attention and sense your surroundings. As your awareness grows, you will develop a new understanding of yourself and others.

Notes

- Visit this book's website at **www.genio.net/pallas**
  where you will find the tide guide, hiker's comments,
  FAQ's, and guided hikes with the author.

- As of April 2003, "trail camping" costs $5.OO/person/night

- **Children age 16 years and under camp free on the trail**
  when with an adult 17 years or older.

- BC Parks allows only paid vehicle camping at Parkinson Crk.
  For wilderness camping, use the Payzant Creek campground
  located 3 Km. west of Parkinson Creek trailhead.

- Enjoy camping at the China Beach tent and RV campground.

- Go to BC Parks website for more information, and current
  camping rates. **wlapwww.gov.bc.ca/bcparks**
  or phone Sooke Museum Info Centre 1-250-642-6351

- Visit **Eagle-Eye Wilderness Company** in Sooke located
  behind the Chevron Gas Station near Sooke town centre for
  camping equipment and tide guides. **www.eagle-eye.ca**

- Special link : **http://www.eagle-eye.ca/mills/mills.htm**

Appendix

Tourist Information Centers

Sooke Regional Museum and Visitor Info. Centre	1-250-642-6351
West Shore Chamber of Commerce (Langford)	1-250-478-1130
BC Parks, South Vancouver Island	1-250-391-2300

Transportation Services To Vancouver Island

Washington State Ferries (Seattle to Victoria)	1-250-382-8100
BC Ferries (Vancouver to Victoria)	1-250-386-3431
Hanna Air Charters (Vancouver to Victoria)	1-800-665-2359
Helijet Airways Inc. (Vancouver to Victoria)	1-250-382-6222
Harbour Air Seaplanes (Vancouver to Victoria)	1-250-384-2215

Transportation Services for the Trail

West Coast Trail Express Bus	1-250-477-8700
(website www.trailbus.com)	
Juan de Fuca Express Jet Boat	1-250-722-2972

Other Unique Local Services

Eagle-Eye Wilderness Co., Sooke, B.C.	1-250-642-7983
(hiking, fishing, and camping equipment)	
& fishing charters)	
Trailhead Resort, Port Renfrew	1-250-647-5468
(rooms, camping, store, charters)	
West Coast Trail Motel, Port Renfrew	1-250-647-5565
(rooms, hot tub, BBQs)	
Lighthouse Pub, Port Renfrew	1-250-647-5505
(restaurant, and pub)	
Shakey's Drive Inn, Jordan River	1-250-646-2184
(outdoor restaurant)	
Explore Charters / On The Sea B&B, Sooke, B.C.	1-250-642-6669
(sailing charters, B&B on an 80 ft. sail boat)	

Emergency and Rescue

Camp Check (hiker's safety service)	1-250-642-2820
Sooke Search and Rescue (Contact R.C.M.P.)	911

Conversions

1 kilometre = 0.62 miles
1 metre = 3.28 feet

For additional maps @ $5.00 each,

write or e-mail to:

Pallas*Trine Services
P.O. Box 137
Sooke, B.C., Canada
V0S 1N0
E-mail: pallas@islandnet.com

*Note: See the updated location of Km. 22 on the map in Chapter 5
entitled "Unmarked Side Trail #4, Chin Beach at Km. 21". See Page 58.*